WHAT SOME HEALTH EXPERTS ARE SAYING ABOUT PAUL NISON'S
RAW KNOWLEDGE

"As in the same vein as his previous book, Paul Nison in a down to earth manner, based mostly on his own experiences and corroborated by a thorough research enthusiastically conveys the importance of a raw diet and a sensible lifestyle. A book that should be on the shelves of every truth seeker."
—**Morris Krok**, Author and long time health authority

"Once again, Paul Nison has given humanity a great gift—his new book, *Raw Knowledge: Enhance the Powers of Your Mind, Body and Soul* —a great, inspiring work about nutrition and health. If one had the conviction and will power necessary to follow Nison's advice and guidelines faithfully, most certainly he/she wouldn't need the services of doctors any longer. Well done Paul."
—**Benito De Donno**, Author of *Glimpses of Reality*

"Paul Nison does it again! Using his own unique sense of wit and wisdom, he creates in his new book, *Raw Knowledge*, an adventure into a land of raw truth and freedom. Paul is so dedicated to his own lifestyle and this dedication is reflected in his books, his lectures and his relationships. I would highly recommend *Raw Knowledge* and suggest that if you ever get a chance to hear Paul in person, go see him. He is a delightful and entertaining speaker full of knowledge and caring for all of life."
—**Roe Gallo** M.A., Author of *Perfect Body*.

"In the entire health education arena, Paul Nison stands out in my mind as being in a special group of the most dynamic, truthful leaders, which I call the *"Raw Passion Gang."* Paul has joined the ranks of true health and self-empowerment teachers, carrying the torch

onward. Paul exudes uncommon dedication toward helping people overcome suffering and mediocre health so that they can get their chance to enjoy life to its fullest. I endorse Paul's books, and refer health truth seekers to his lectures and seminars, because from Paul they will get a real caring person and a liberating, insight-filled, exuberant experience."
—**David Klein**, Creator of *Raw Passion Seminars*, Publisher of *Living Nutrition Magazine*, Director of *Colitis & Crohn's Health Recovery Services*, Co-founder of *Healthful Living International*.

"There will never be enough people like Paul Nison on this planet! The world needs the message from the *Raw Life*. I fully support your work and your ideas."
—**Frederic Patenaude**, Publisher of *Just Eat An Apple Magazine* and author of *Sunfood Cuisine*.

"Time's a-wasting! If you're tired of feeling tired, sick of being sick, and resist being prescribed drugs to merely treat symptoms with no attempt to get at the cause, you are ready to do what's prescribed in this book! I'm convinced that if people just knew the powerful effects in store for them with this dietary change, they'd get mad that nobody told them sooner!"
—**Ruth Heidrich**, Ph.D., Ironman Triathlete.

"*Raw Knowledge* by Paul Nison suggests a way that can make a meaningful contribution to overcoming disease, upgrading health and enjoying life more. This book testifies to the indisputable benefits of a raw diet. It is fascinating and is written with an inner conviction which will touch you. It is for everyone who wants to live a healthy and happy life."
—Professor **Célène Bernstein**, Author of *Health Seekers*.

"Paul Nison is an outstanding vibration of the emerging generation of raw and living foodists. As one who has been on the raw and living foods scene for several decades, I am personally gratified to see this young man arise from a raw and living foods student to take a strong leadership role in the growing raw and living foods move-

ment. This book is definitely key for those who are striving to gain a greater conceptual understanding of a holistic living way of life through the divine consumption of raw and living foods."
—**High Priest Kwatamani**, Author and life empowerment speaker,
www.livefoodsunchild.com

"As Henry David Thoreau (American philosopher) once said, "Being is the great explainer." Paul takes these words to heart by presenting an inspiring, rare peek into the lives of fellow raw foodists. Through his signature uplifting, non-threatening manner, the reader can easily glean valuable 'Raw-Food Lifestyle' information and/or choose points which bear further personal investigation! *Rawsome*! Although Paul teaches from the heart of his own personal experience, he humbly embraces the knowledge of other raw foodists as well. His 'livi'cation and humor is beautifully reflected within, warmly inviting all to understand the beneficial truths behind raw food consumption and the many paths which lead to experiencing them."
—**Karen Fierro**, BFA, LMT, CYI, *www.GardenOfHealth.com*

"No one but Paul Nison could have written this book. His unique slant on life touches a common chord within us all. We cannot help but agreeing with him, and loving him for showing us his insights. It takes a special someone to rise up from the crowd and create something unique. Paul Nison is just such a someone. He is changing the world. With the creation of his first book, *The Raw Life*, he became a known entity in the raw world. Now, three years later, Paul Nison has shown that he is no flash in the pan, but is a leader that is here to stay. He has created another winner with his new book, *Raw Knowledge*. Like Paul himself, this book is unpretentious and worth spending time with. It is something that only Paul Nison could have created, and I am very glad he did. As you learn more of Paul's philosophy on life, you will find that succeeding on raw will become easier for you. Read the interviews with many of the world's most successful raw fooders and learn *Raw Knowledge*."
—**Dr. Douglas N. Graham**, Author of *The High Energy Diet Recipe Guide*, *Nutrition and Athletic Performance*, *Grain Damage*, *Hygienic Fasting* and *Perpetual Health*.

RAW KNOWLEDGE, Part II

Interviews with Health Achievers

Paul Nison

343 Publishing Company
Brooklyn, New York

Disclaimer:

This book is not intended as medical advice. When going on a natural diet, there is always some risk involved. Because of this, the author, publisher and /or distributors of this book are not responsible for any adverse detoxification effects or consequences resulting from the use of any suggestions or procedures described herein.

This book is printed on recycled paper.

Art direction and design: Enrique Candioti
Cover illustration: Sunstar
All other illustrations: Tom Cushwa
Editor: Joel Brody

Library of Congress Catalog Card Number: 2001118701

ISBN # 0-9675286-2-3

Copyright @ 2003 by Paul Nison

First edition January, 2003

All rights reserved. No part of this book may be reproduced, by any means, except for brief quotations embodied in articles and reviews, without the written consent from the author.

343 Publishing Company
PO Box 443
Brooklyn NY 11209

Paul Nison is also the author of:

The Raw Life: Becoming Natural in an Unnatural World
Raw Knowledge: Enhance the Powers of Your Mind, Body and Soul
Raw Life: Achieving Your Goals (compact disc)
The Raw Life (audio tape series)

Dedication

This book is dedicated to my good friend, Dr. Fred Bisci. Fred, thanks for sharing your knowledge with me and so many others. I will never forget the lessons you continue to teach me. If everyone had a friend and teacher like you, this world would be a better place.

Acknowledgements

I'd like to thank everyone who has helped me with this book and my raw life journey. I've made many good friends. We may not speak everyday, but you are in my mind all the time. You're all very special to me, my raw family, giving me support and teaching me great lessons about health, trust, life, happiness, love, freedom and success. Some of you have welcomed me into your homes when you didn't even know me because I needed a place to stay. I will never forget your hospitality. Thank you, thank you, thank you.

I'd also like to thank everyone who has helped me put this book together. We worked hard, but all our hard work has been rewarded, because now it's done. Thank you all so much for helping me get my message out and helping others. You are all so special to me:

Dave Norman, Fred Bisci, Tom Cushwa, Enrique Candioti, Joel Brody and an extra special thanks to Amy Yockel. Amy you are a modern day Peace Pilgrim.

Thanks to everyone I interviewed for this book or Part One of this book: Annette Larkins, Celene Bernstein, Roz Gruben, Essie Haniball, The High Priest Kofi Kwatamani and Kwatamani family community; Viktoras Kulvinskas, Youkta, Gabriel Cousens, William Esser, Renée Loux Underkoffler, Ruth Heidrich, Annie Jubb, Katherine Clark, Karen Fierro, Rhio and Leih, Dave Klein, Arne Wingqvist, John Fielder, Robert Sniadach, Arthur Andrews and Dr. V. Virginia Vetrano.

And my thanks go to everyone who has bought this book. You've given me support in continuing to help spread the message of life empowerment. You give what you get, so keep giving support and you will keep receiving support in return.

Contents

DEDICATION	viii
ACKNOWLEDGEMENTS	ix
A WORD FROM THE AUTHOR	13
INTRODUCTION	15

The INTERVIEWS	23
Karen Fierro	27
Katharine Clark	45
Ruth Heidrich	63
Renée Loux Underkoffler	73
Rhio	89
Annie Jubb	103

Contents

Arne Wingqvist	115
David Klein	141
Robert Sniadach	159
John Fielder	177
Arthur Andrews	191
Dr. V. Virginia Vetrano	209
Paul Nison	251
CONCLUSION	263
About the Author	271
Raw Support: Support the Raw Life	277

A Word from the Author

How much food do you need to be healthy? Is there a cure for all diseases? How much sleep do you need every night? How can you be at your best mentally, physically and spiritually? What will keep you happy all the time? How can you be free?

Where can all the answers be found to so many questions? You can start by reading *Raw Knowledge: Enhance the Powers of Your Mind, Body and Soul*. This book is the continuation to that book. But the order in which you read them really doesn't matter. Read them both to be enlightened with many answers to these questions.

I received all the information in these books from the people I interviewed. Unlike the common people on the street, these people are special - leaders of their own lives. They've decided not to be like the common person and do the common thing just because it makes "common sense" or because it's the popular thing to do. Instead, they've decided to listen to their own "body sense." Despite what anyone else thought or said, they did, and continue to do, what feels best to them.

They are leaders. They have the answers. And now their answers are available to you. These answers cannot be ignored if you want to be the best you can be. If you want to tap into your body's own special, innate powers, read their messages, messages for success. Their interviews will help you achieve your goals, motivate you to put your dreams into action, turning them into reality.

I'm so excited to present this information to you and I thank you for your support in buying this book.

Introduction

This book is a continuation of *Raw Knowledge, Part I: Enhance the Powers of Your Mind, Body and Soul*. Part One contains important information to help you learn and grow. When I decided to write *Raw Knowledge*, my idea was to include many interviews with people who have been successful in achieving their goals, becoming the best they could be, mentally, physically and emotionally. I achieved this idea. All of the people I interviewed had several major experiences in common. On the topic of diet, they all ate mostly uncooked, natural foods. Many of them have been successful at eating an all raw vegan diet for many years. Many people today think it must be very hard to eat a diet of only raw food. The people I've interviewed prove all doubters wrong. It can be done, and all the subjects of my interviews have done it. Natural foods, eaten raw, have kept their bodies and minds in optimal working order. Although some of them are far older than the common young sick person today, they're much healthier and happier than most common people today on the poor common diet. Do you see the connection? The people I interviewed have seen the connection for a long time and explain it in their interviews.

Another understanding all the subjects of the interviews had in common was that although all humans are built the same, with the exception of some minor hereditary traits, no two people are in the same place at the same time. What might work for one person might not work for another "at this time." But as long as everyone keeps cleaning his/her mind, body and soul, he/she will reach the same place of excellent health and happiness. The experts I interviewed have long understood the importance of not only putting natural,

Introduction

unprocessed food into their bodies, but also to feed their minds with good, positive thoughts. What you put in is what you get out, and what you put out is what you get in. It's a cycle that has continued to happen until today and will continue to happen always.

What have I learned from all the people I've met and interviewed over the years?

It all starts in the mind. Our belief system is formed at an early age. We're conditioned to do certain things and think a certain way. We're conditioned to follow, rather than to lead. We're conditioned to do the most popular thing, not the most sensible thing. We listen to common sense, not body sense. Before you can enhance the power of your mind, you must first un-condition yourself: un-learn before you can learn. It all starts in the mind.

The cleaner the mind, the easier it will be to clean the body. The more knowledge you gather as to what foods are best for the body, the less fear you'll suffer in the face of commonly held false pronouncements about diet and health. More knowledge equals less fear. Fear dwells in going against popular or commonly held beliefs. Knowledge is the foundation of success and becoming a leader, a trailblazer. What others are doing is not important. Know thyself and understand your own body.

Once the mind and body are clean, you will experience a clean soul. There is a whole world out there that is hidden to the eyes of the owner of a mind and body that are not clean. Once cleaned, you will see a whole new beautiful world.

Put good energy out, and that is what you will receive. There are two sets of laws: laws made by governments and laws of nature. Government laws are laws people are told they must follow or else. But government laws don't include the understanding of karma and the cosmic laws of the universe. Government laws only focus on the outcome without paying any attention to the intent; whereas cosmic laws are those we are not told to live by, but laws we feel are natural and want to live by. Cosmic laws don't focus on outcome, but instead focus on intent. Have good intentions and the outcome will be good, no matter how it appears. Sometimes something will happen and people won't understand why, but everything happens for a reason and when the time is right, we will find out that reason. Sometimes things happen that might seem bad, but turn out well - blessings in disguise.

Some major keys to success are found below in a list that can go on and on. If you want to eat an all raw diet or achieve anything else in life, it's possible, easy and you can do it. There are no limits to the number of keys to success you can have. The more keys you have, the more answers you'll receive. Keep learning, keep growing. Keep moving forward. No limits!

a) Never accept anything less than the best for yourself. Don't leave yourself any other possible outcome. Many unsuccessful people leave themselves only two possible outcomes: bad or worse; and they'll settle for bad. How many times have you heard people say with satisfaction, "It could have been worse." They will accept a 'bad' outcome. Instead, leave yourself only these two outcomes: good or better. Your willingness to accept only these two outcomes will guarantee you a positive outcome.

b) Have an open mind. Don't limit yourself to any beliefs. Never say never. One of the major keys to success is to have an open mind. The more open you are to trying new things in life that make sense to you, the more you will find new answers. If you limit your knowledge, you limit your life. Remember: NO LIMITS!

c) There is no such thing as being selfish. Many people today

Introduction

place the needs of others before their own. They go out of their way to help others while hurting themselves in the process. People take advantage of you when they see how much they can get from you. They get used to it, and once you don't put their needs before yours, they call you selfish. This makes a nice person feel guilty. It's a trap. There is no such thing as selfish. If there were, the only person who is truly selfish is the person getting upset and calling you selfish because you weren't putting his needs before your own. Put yourself first. Make yourself happy FIRST. Let others take care of themselves and worry about themselves. Once you've achieved what you want and you are content, then is the time to help others. But to continue to help others while neglecting your own health and happiness is to set yourself up for failure and an unfulfilled life.

d) Live every day as if it's your last moment. You can buy many things in life, but time is one thing you cannot buy. To waste any precious moment of your life is simply wasting your own life. Why put things off till tomorrow if you are here and can do them today. "Because I don't have time," you say. Well, make the time! You're worth it. No excuses. Use your time wisely. There are many ways people waste time, but today's major time waster is watching television programming. If you want to add a lot of extra time to your life, the first thing to do is to throw away your television set. Most people are addicted to television programming and would immediately think there is no way they could live without a TV set in their homes. If this is the way you're thinking, you're wasting time. Throw it out and see how much more time you gain in your life. With all that extra time, fulfill your dreams. Make them a reality.

e) Keep it simple; less is more. Many people go through life trying to get as many material items as possible, thinking that the more they own the better off they are. This is not true, in fact, if you own too many things, your things will own you. The only thing you should seek to obtain much of is knowledge. Store it in the mind. Doing so will leave you burden free. The fewer items you possess, the more freedom you have to go wherever you want and do whatever you want to do. Learn the difference between a want and a need. Limit the items you choose to those you must have and truly need. You shouldn't want more than you need. It's okay to have certain items that you don't truly need, but enjoy, but limit them, as too many at one time can also complicate your life. Need it, use it, enjoy it and then, when you are finished with it, pass it on to someone who needs it more than you.

f) Have passion! Do only those things you enjoy in life, in work, and in everything. Doing things that you don't enjoy not only wastes your time, but also causes damage to your mind and body. There is a great way to know if you really enjoy something. When you're doing it, are you able to smile? If so, then you're enjoying your passion in life, and you're on the road to achieving your goals. However, if you're having a hard time smiling and enjoying what you're doing, change it at once, or the outcome will be fatal. From work, to diet, to relationships and everything else, if you're not enjoying it, stop it. Don't waste time trying to change it, just stop it, and move on to something else that you do enjoy.

g) It's okay to say no. Most people feel guilty saying no. It's okay to tell people no, if that's how you feel. If they can't accept your answer, that's their problem, not yours. There is no need to have to waste time explaining your "no" response to anyone. Let them deal with it and move on. You don't owe anyone an excuse ever! Spending time giving people excuses

Introduction

is just wasting your valuable time. There is no excuse for that.

h) Keep moving forward! The body and the mind never stand still. The body and the mind are always moving, either forward or backwards. There is no such thing as standing still. You must keep moving forward always. It's okay to slow down if you feel you're going too fast, but don't stop. Keep moving in the right direction and you will achieve success.

i) Be confident! Disregard any negative information people might give you. You can achieve your goals no matter what they are. There are no limits to what you can achieve as long as you're confident.

j) Take action! There are dreamers and there are doers. It's good to set goals and dream about achieving them, but they won't come true if you don't take action on them. Don't wait for them to happen; make them happen!

k) Be FREE! This is what it all comes down to: being free in an unfree world, free to be the best you can be. Learn what freedom really is, and set yourself up to be as free as you can possibly be. Freedom gives you the power and tools you will need to achieve your goals.

l) Get whatever you want! Become the person you want to be! Relax, visualize and believe. These three things will help you create and obtain anything you want in life. First you must relax and get control of your emotions; next you must visualize where you want to be and who you want to be. Don't ask yourself, "What can I get?" Ask yourself, "What can I become?" Don't think about it as, "I will become," think of it as "I am." Don't think of how it feels to want something, think of how it feels to have it now. Live in the now. Visualize how it

Introduction

feels, and then believe! Believe in yourself, not that you can obtain it, but instead think that you've already obtained it. Relaxing, visualizing and believing in yourself will get you whatever you want in life.

m) To keep it, be thankful! You can have all you want. Creating it and getting it is easy, as long as you relax, visualize and believe. But it can go away just as fast if you're not thankful for it. Be thankful for all that you have gotten, and you will keep it. As soon as you stop being thankful, it all goes away just as fast as it came.

n) Keep seeking knowledge: from this book, these interviews, all the educational opportunities around you. The lessons are there and waiting. Go and get them; and never stop moving forward, enhancing the powers of your mind, body and soul.

These major keys to success will help you clean your mind. Once your mind is clean, it will be easy to clean your body. Once your body is clean, you'll truly be able to deal with or experience the beauty of spirituality. Keep enhancing, keep growing, and keep moving forward. There are no limits to what you can do. Diet is a very important step, but the body works as a whole, in mind, body and soul. You must nourish and enhance all of them equally. Most important: you much enjoy the journey of life.

"Life without leaning is death." -Unknown

The Interviews

This book continues in the same vein as my first two books, *The Raw Life*, and *Raw Knowledge, Part One*, which both contain interviews. These interviews are appreciated by many readers because there is something in them for everyone. Not every reader will connect with all the men and women who were the subjects of these interviews, but there is always something an expert says that will make sense to a reader. Do only what makes sense to you, no matter who says it. If it doesn't make sense to you, don't even attempt it.

After examining the interviews in my first two books, many readers were confused because I asked the subjects exactly the same questions and got completely opposite answers. People asked me, "Who is right and who is wrong?" All of them are right. Nothing they said and did is wrong. No two people are in the same place at the same time, and they each did what worked best for them at that time in their lives. You, too, must do what makes sense to you at this particular time in your life. Do it! If it works, great. If you give it enough time

The Interviews

and it doesn't work, then do something else. If you keep doing something that continues to produce an undesirable result, you must change it if you want a different and desirable result. Have fun, and find what works best for you.

Enjoy these interviews. In future editions of this book, I will be adding more interviews with experts I meet on my path. I will also update some of these interviews. As their subjects find new information, their responses may change at some future time. Keep in touch, either through my website:

www.rawlife.com

or call me at:

866-RAW-DIET (866-729-3438)

or by mail:

Paul Nison
P.O. Box 443
Brooklyn, NY 11209

*Note that as I move in the future, this mailing address might change. You may view updated information on my website, or call the toll free number that will remain the same.

I'd love you to keep in touch with me and give me an update on how well you're doing. Also, please help me to help others. Share your success story with me, even before and after pictures, if you like, that I can add to my website or a future book. I look forward to hearing from you. Enjoy these interviews.

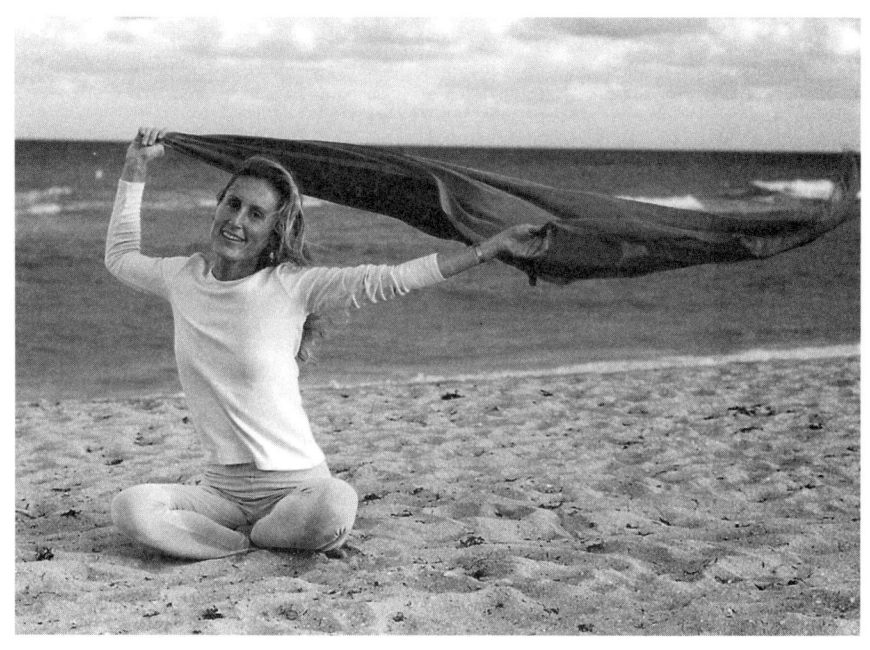

You may contact Karen at:

Web Site: www.gardenofhealth.com
Email: Karen@gardenofhealth.com
Miami-Live: 305-672-5878

Karen Fierro

Karen's interest in natural health and Yoga began eighteen years ago. After receiving a BFA from Parsons School of Design and The New School for Social Research in New York, she incorporated vegetarian dietary standards into her lifestyle. She worked in several New York City museums and co-directed the Department of Ceramics at Brooklyn College, Brooklyn, N.Y. In Manhattan, she met vegetarian-Natural Hygiene advocate, Peter E. Firk and renowned author-lecturer Viktoras Kulvinskas, M.S. Karen was invited to contribute her research and artistic talents to their joint venture known as *The Vegetarian Lifestyle Home & Travel Guide*, becoming Assistant Production Manager from 1990 to 1999. The Guide soon found an expanded home on the internet in 1999 as www.VegetarianUSA.com where it has received over 10,000,000 hits.

Over the years she developed and maintained good working relationships with many key professional members of the Natural Hygiene, Raw and Living Food communities. Independent study of nutrition and Yoga amplified her desire to educate the general public on important health issues. From 1991 to 1992 she successfully co-directed the New Haven Vegetarian Society in New Haven, CT. From 1993 to 1995 she co-founded and subsequently co-directed the Miami Vegetarian Society in Miami, FL and from 2000-2003 directed/created the first Living Food Support group in South Florida called Miami-Live! In December of 2000 she produced a Natural Hygiene/Living Food educational website called www.GardenOfHealth.com which has received over 300,000 hits since opening.

In 1994, she became a Licensed Massage Therapist in Miami, FL., followed by a one year stay as Research Consultant with the pioneering Touch Research Institute (T.R.I.), University of Miami, Jackson Memorial Hospital. She directed four studies on the effects of massage therapy with chronic fatigue, fibromyalgia, eating disorders and spousal abuse patients. Budgetary cuts interrupted completion of three but fibromyalgia was finalized and later published in the *Journal of Clinical Rheumatology* 2, 18-22. 1996. During this time her Massage Therapy practice flourished while upholding her responsibilities www.VegetarianUSA.com.

In November, 1999 she achieved certification as a Sampoorna Yoga Instructor (a form based on Sivananda style). Practice of Vipassana meditation and TM is ongoing, coupled with attending special nationwide retreat programs.

Currently Karen resides in Miami Beach, Florida. Her lifestyle centers around practicing massage therapy, teaching yoga, freelance graphic design, fine art (painting), live-food lifestyle consultation, organic gardening, fun and sunshine.

When did you first hear about the raw food diet, and what made you want to try it?
About eighteen years ago, I was introduced to the concept of uncooked food consumption by Barbara Feldman, a Natural Fertility Awareness specialist in New York City. She invited me to her annual New Year's Eve Raw Food Potluck Party, and out of curiosity, I accepted. On reflection, the idea of a full dinner consisting of 'raw food' was so foreign to my awareness, Barbara literally had to advise me on what to bring! There I met Peter E. Firk, Essene, Natural Hygienist and Director of www.VegetarianUSA.com. A romance blossomed, and through the grace of his careful Essene guidance, I learned in greater depth about the many realms within this lifestyle which we practiced together. This marked the first phase in my living food transition. Without a doubt, when I learned about the heightened spiritual attunement which occurs after consistent live food consumption, I was interested in trying it.

How was your health before you started the diet?
Although I would have said it was great eighteen years ago when I was consuming standard American fare, I have come to learn that warning flags were flying high regarding inappropriate physical care. I suffered from chronic constipation since early childhood and into my early 20s. In fact, I believed it was a normal part of adulthood! Another significant indication was relentless physical lethargy. This troublesome dilemma proved to be a blessing in disguise, for it prompted me to analyze lifestyle habits with greater scrutiny.

How long did it take you to heal once you started eating a raw food diet?
When I transitioned to standard vegetarian, energy improved and the constipation lessened. During this period colonic irrigation was included on a few occasions as well. But when the amount of living food was increased, eventually to a high degree over the span of a year or two, healing of these symptoms was brought all the way to the finish line! In fact, I remember being so overjoyed with the ease and amount of my evacuations that I exuberantly announced it to anyone who was in earshot of the bathroom! A lifetime of physical constriction and agony had been miraculously erased.

When you tried this diet for the first time, what attracted you to it?
The heightened spiritual attunement with the natural world attracted me. All the other benefits unfurled over time as unexpected bonus prizes. But after the first three years of about 70% to 90% raw, progress on the path slowed as my work and lifestyle responsibilities increased. The percentage of raw consumption dropped significantly and fluctuated like a roller coaster year after year. What remained clear was an inner resolve to eventually get back to a diet that included a higher and more consistent level of living food. Years later,

this resolve began to manifest but with one big difference. This time my focus was to learn more about how to embrace the diet through all aspects of human experience (emotional stress, workplace influences, high physical output, etc.). With the addition of juice cleansing, a few more recipes, study, and communication with other Natural Hygienists and Living Foodists, the process became more practical. Herein marked the second phase of my living food transition which began about 11 years ago and has been wonderfully evolving since.

It sounds like Peter was a big inspiration to you. Are you and Peter still a couple?
Peter and I amicably ended our nine and a half year partnership five years ago, yet we still remain as close friends in support of one another's higher aspirations.

Who inspired you the most to eat a raw food diet?
Narrowing it down, I'd have to say five people. Number one was Peter E. Firk, who back in 1985 introduced me to this lifestyle in marvelous depth. It was through him that I adopted an understanding of the pure lifestyle practices of the Ancient Essenes and more! Two others were our friends, Lenny Watson and his girlfriend at the time, Damaris. Their system of living a raw food lifestyle was unlike anything I had ever seen til then. Cases of sub-tropical produce in the dining room and kitchen, pitchers full of fresh pressed juice, freshly made raw dressings and pre-cut salad greens in the fridge, three to four jumbo jars of seeds and legumes sprouting over the kitchen sink at any given time...The fragrant alive aroma from within their home was amazing, not to mention their glowing appearance and vitality. Then, in 1998, I entrusted Dr. Doug Graham to take me on as a fasting patient. At his former Marathon, Florida home, I underwent a Hygienic Fast for fourteen days, soon after building-up, cross-training, consulting, and fine-tuning my approach to living food preparation. My commitment deepened on all levels. Of recent date, I have

been abundantly blessed to meet High Priest Kwatamani. If I were asked to name a spiritual leader within the living food movement, it would be this very developed soul. His presence, service, insight and clarity reveal the deeply profound, seldomly elaborated truths. I thank him and his divine family for their example, love and encouragement!

You've learned so much over the years. What are some of the most important things you've learned?
We know that the growth of a plant is dependent upon the integrity of the seed, soil conditions, water, climate, sunshine, interaction from the natural world and so on. When all factors are intact, the plant thrives and gives abundantly. Humans are no different. Our bodies depend upon sunshine, clean environment, fresh food from the garden, pure water to cleanse outer and inner body, interaction with nature and much more. Living food consumption is invaluable because the body's chemistry, sensory awareness, inherent spiritual affinity, physical beauty and efficiency, emotional stability, (etc.) are given the opportunity to be fully expressed. But it is wise to be patient with transitioning. The dogma of "doing it right all the time no matter what" can lead to great struggle and stress. Doing your best then slipping off the path from time to time is part of the process. I, for one, have done so repeatedly over the years, at times diving into pasta, vegetarian Thai, breads, potato chips, vegetarian pizza... my old comfort foods. But after the initial flavor burst and feast, the change inevitably becomes very disappointing. It never feels the same as I remembered, because mind, body and emotions have been exposed to a much more refined way. Directly experiencing the large and subtle differences can be a powerful learning tool! That is why it is *essential* to support a positive mental focus by commiserating with like-minded health seekers, utilizing living food resources such as books, videos, audio and internet, participate in workshops or events, purchase or grow

high quality organic foods when possible, meditate, incorporate Live Organic Juice Cleanses, better still, Guided Hygienic Fasting. But if a person is faced with life threatening illness and chooses to incorporate living foods, I highly recommend they seek the guidance of a Natural Hygiene Consultant or Living Foods Health Center to help determine the correct approach and pace.

Are there any pitfalls you have learned to watch out for on the raw diet?
Well, for nearly half my life, food choices revolved around the salty-sweet flavors found in cooked dishes. Tongue in cheek, I was a member of Salt Addicts Anonymous! In the beginning of my transition, it was inconceivable to cease using processed salt so I upgraded my choices to *Braggs Liquid Aminos, low sodium Tamari, Celtic sea salt, or Herbamare and stayed with them for many years. Herein lies the importance and beauty of Hygienic Fasting. After the June 2001, ten day fast I deeply realized that this seemingly irresistible lure was revealed to be an obstacle, as I continue to move towards a more consistent living food consumption pattern. Even the attraction to cooked food is due in great measure to processed salt for without it, cooked food tastes dead. It is also the catalyst of many negative symptoms, including quick temper, over anxiousness, caffeine-like speediness and subsequent energy drop, drier skin, joint stiffness/achiness, puffiness in face and body, extra thirst, and the desire to consume concentrated sweet foods. So I add celery or celery juice to raw dishes or enjoy them as they are. It just feels better all around!

The other most common challenges I've faced are travel, socializing, and a busy schedule. Here are some simple solutions for them:

*Important note: of recent date, Braggs has come under great scrutiny by the Natural Hygiene community regarding how it is processed and its composition. To learn more, contact Healthful Living International.

1) Always have food with you when going about your daily schedule such as nuts, seeds, nut butter, and fruit. When possible, consume thick frozen banana or other fruit smoothies between meals.

2) Shop in the grocery store on a full stomach.

3) The quantity of living food consumed by a living foodist is typically more than our mainstream friends, families, or restaurants will serve. So when dining out, consume a satiating living food meal just *before* arriving.

4) Travel? Be sure to pack in your carry-on luggage avocados, nut butter, tahini, resilient fruit, salad greens in a reusable bag, water, etc. If you are staying in a hotel outside a major city, add to your luggage a portable blender, eating utensils, a bowl, and a small chopping board. When you arrive, find the nearest health food store or major supermarket and stock up.

5) When possible, purchase the *highest* quality raw organic food available. When ingredients are of greatest nutrient value and freshness, the desire for cooked food diminishes. Yes, it may cost a bit more, but it is well worth it to feel really satisfied and on-track. I purchase nuts, seeds, and nut butters from mail-order sources, grow my own organic produce or (a few times/month) buy bulk freshly-picked organic produce from a farm to supplement what I typically buy from local stores.

Dental problems are another big pitfall. Do you have any thoughts about that?
When I over-rely on high acid fruit such as oranges, grapefruit, and pineapple, my dental weak-links make themselves known. So rather than create a potential problem, I consume

a variety of nutrients by incorporating a diverse range of organic produce, nuts and seeds each week. My enjoyment of citrus is in no way hampered, but consumption is regulated a bit more. Although a good dental evaluation is definitely on the agenda, it is comforting to know that at least for now, I am able to keep these weak-links at bay.

What do you think about mercury fillings, and what would you replace them with?
Certainly, replacing mercury fillings should be on everyone's list of important things to do for health. It's a good idea to research what modern dentistry has come up with in recent years, as new and better compounds become available.

What is your opinion of nuts and seeds?
They are excellent natural sources of protein and essential fatty acids. They contain lecithin and B-vitamins and are rich sources of minerals. They also supply necessary bulk in the diet. Soak them before using, and always try to buy high quality organic.

What is your opinion of grains?
Sprouted or soaked grain salads can offer a different taste and texture excursion, but for me they tend to bring on thirst, often times flatulence after eating. So I visit this dining experience on rare occasions.

What is your opinion of fruitarianism?
Over the years, I have observed many who consume fruit exclusively. Signs of physical degeneration were evident. That is why I advocate a well-rounded diet that includes raw nuts, seeds, sprouted legumes, and leafy veggies. The elements within these fuel sources are relevant to the overall maintenance of the body. One who consumes a high to 100% living food diet is typically taking in mostly fruit in conjunction with these, anyway.

What is your opinion of sprouts?
A wonderful way to consume organic legumes or seeds.

What is your opinion of Natural Hygiene?
It offers predominantly accurate, sound health information, great stuff! But to be better accepted by today's standards NH's scope must embrace more: in my opinion, female issues, organic back-to-the-land living (growing), environment, healing modalities including: massage therapy, colonic irrigation, juice cleansing, the use of Yoga and biggest of all...Spirituality. Over the years, I've always selected the best each area has to offer, when appropriate. Luckily, Healthful Living International, Transformational Institute and Living Nutrition Magazine are expanding NH's definition to embrace a more complete holistic picture. I highly support them!

What is your opinion of supplements?
Supplements are isolated elements which have been chemically extracted. Less evidence exists to substantiate the effectiveness of supplements as opposed to what has been proven to be beneficial within whole fruits and veggies where thousands of phytochemicals (many not yet identified by contemporary science) exist to specifically and readily absorb into the human body. Devoid of life energy, pills or potions could never grow if planted in the ground no matter how ideal the conditions. But if one is concerned about getting proper nutrition, it may be prudent to get a scientific nutritional analysis and work with a Natural Hygiene Consultant to determine the best approach. Society's reliance on supplements, algaes included, is counter-productive to the well being of our plane, since the process of manufacturing them creates factory pollution, uses synthetic substances, materials and exploited labor. I feel it is of extreme importance to support organic agriculture and especially cooperative organic agriculture (equal work, equal pay). Let us improve the freshness, inher-

ent nutrition, human fairness and cost effectiveness so organically grown food is not just for the elite, but becomes the norm for everyone regardless of income level.

What is your opinion of eating seasonally?
Personally, I enjoy and find greater nutritional value in variety. I like to buy locally grown organic produce as much as possible throughout the year and grow what I can. This, coupled with what my local market brings in from other parts of the country, makes for something of a balance. "Adapt, adjust, and accommodate" is something a great spiritual teacher I admire once said.

What is your opinion of fasting?
An extremely beneficial modality! It has been an invaluable tool in helping me to deeply understand my emotional and physical attraction to certain foods with lasting results. Guided Hygienic Fasting provides the body with the deep rest, repair, detoxification, and rejuvenation it needs. After my fasts, the desire for higher food choices increased and the benefit list is LONG. It's remarkable to witness the power and wisdom the human body possesses to self-heal! The fasting process traverses through sometimes rough, other times peaceful terrain. That is why it is highly recommended that a doctor specializing in Hygienic Fasting be on hand to first assess if one is ready, then assist along the way.

What is your opinion of food combining on a 100% raw diet, and is it necessary?
Here again, I speak from my own experience. I have found it's extremely beneficial to learn the principles of Food Combining. It has acted as a very clear guide in helping me to understand why I felt uncomfortable after one meal and not another. Proper Food Combining makes for easier digestion and a better emotional disposition for sure. However, in some instances I am able to consume a combination or two which

might be considered inappropriate with light side effects. That is why I feel that although the principles are very sound, it is still something each individual must decipher for him or herself. After many years, this awareness continues to evolve as my body changes.

What is your opinion of physical exercise?
A great essential for health and an exceptionally important chapter in the owners manual of the human body!

What is your opinion of wild foods?
With keen awareness in distinguishing poisonous from non-poisonous, delicious from bitter, wild foods are extremely powerful food choices.

What are your age, height, and weight? Has your weight changed, or were there any other changes your body went through? How did you handle it?
My current age is forty. To honor this body, I celebrated with a ten-day Hygienic Water Fast in June of 2001. I look at it this way. If fasting is a tool which can help add time onto one's lifespan, help maintain a youthful appearance, and offer a better chance at living many more years in a vital manner, then it's truly a small price to pay. My height is still 5'6" and my weight is 112 pounds. As I overview these transitional years, it is indeed true that higher amounts of living food consumption did yield to a gradual reduction in body weight. Here are two other asides. Rather unexpectedly, I found the loss of old-fat hanging on the thighs and buttocks occurred due to my first Guided Hygienic Fast and the exercise, yoga, and active professional life I carried on afterwards. At least eight pounds never returned as I continued with 70% to 100% living food. And when cold pressed (including the best olive oil) or cooked oil was completely omitted, body fat reduced there too and I didn't miss a thing. Because now it was possible to freely enjoy avocado, other fatty fruits, nuts, nut butters, and tahini with

greater frequency, in proper balance with other foods.

Did you ever get really sick or have a really bad detox during your transition to this diet?
I chose a gradual transition over many years (still going on today). It seemed more natural to do it that way, especially since I was not faced with a life-threatening condition. So for the most part, I experienced a minimal number of detoxing symptoms. When I began, Live Organic Juice Cleansing was part of my monthly plan to move the detoxing process along. I called it "cleansing the palette." When nausea or headaches appeared, I took rest until they passed. After all, my body was directly coming from a predominantly cooked vegetarian and before that, standard American diet. These moments were my first big glimpses at understanding how food choices affect body, mind, and emotions.

Do you eat 100% raw foods, and if so, for how long? If not, how much raw food do you eat, and what do you eat that is cooked?
My transitioning process has been evolving and steadily improving over the last eleven years. I will go for months at a time on 90-100%, and then fluctuate for months afterward. When I do, it's typically during periods of very concentrated and intense physical and mental work. Here I try to limit cooked food choices to steamed veggies, baked potato, maybe rice along with salad, fresh fruit and frozen smoothies, nuts and seeds. Sometimes I eat other cooked veggie choices 'out' when prep-time just isn't there, or I'm tired. I'm sure to find the best way to handle these periods with more living food, but for now that's where I'm at. Another challenge is out of town travel. Although I take every measure necessary to stay on track, the unexpected can still happen. If well into a retreat (which usually offers standard vegetarian fare in an institutional setting) or in a remote locale where live foods are in scant supply, personal surplus has dwindled, I go for rice, po-

tato, plain steamed veggies or other plain food. My motto is "do what you can do." For if my disposition is groggy and exhausted instead of up and cheerful, it affects me and those with whom I come in contact. It's all a work in progress.

What is your average daily diet like? What do you eat, and how often?
Average raw-days begin with fruit for breakfast, sometimes in the form of a smoothie, or seasonal fruits until full, or a few fresh coconut pieces washed down with coconut water. Lunch is the biggest meal of the day and can be a large bowl of celery slaw, large salad with salad herbs, tomato, soaked sunflower seeds and raw dressing. I snack on fruit smoothies and nuts between meals. Dinner can be another salad, or a combo of different fruit and veggies with nuts and seeds, sometimes durian, etc. The amount and choice of what to consume at each meal also depends on the kind of activity the day will require. So this "typical day menu" just gives a rough sketch. If I haven't gotten enough variety from the organic produce area of my market, then I will turn to the standard produce area for new choices. Although organic is always number one and still makes up a large percentage of my diet, diversifying maintains a wide range of nutritional support and keeps the menu fun. As often as possible, I purchase organic nuts, seeds, and nut butters through quality mail-order sources. And a few times per month, my friends and I will drive down to an organic farm or two, bringing back whatever fruit is up-for-grabs. For after consuming foods that are grown and/or picked within hours of consumption, I have no curiosity for cooked food when I go out into the world. It makes a huge difference!

What is your favorite food?
When available, my current highlights are English peas, Herb Salad mix, sweet watermelon, durian in season, canistel, Haas avocados, passion fruit, Fuji apples, bananas and pine nuts (as a treat). Those are my favorite foods now, but this could

change over the months.

How are your health and energy?
Both are great!

How much sleep do you get, and how much do you think is necessary?
Oh, when I haven't taken an afternoon nap, it can be seven to eight hours. With an afternoon nap, it can be less. I think each and every human must get a lot of rest to handle what society and our responsibilities call for. We as a society are severely sleep/rest deprived. Skimping on the only time the body gets to repair and rejuvenate destroys health! I don't think one should consider *'sleeping less'* worthy of a badge of honor, unless it *truly* feels perfect.

What mental changes have you noticed?
In one of the oldest health traditions, Yoga, there are three qualities or Gunas. They are Tamasic, Rajasic and Sattvic. Rajasic foods are very hot, bitter, sour, dry, or salty. They disrupt the mind-body equilibrium by stimulating the body and making the mind restless. Tamasic foods include fermented items, stale and rotten items, garlic, onions, and all meat. Tamasic deprives the body of Prana (life energy), creating inertia, and the powers of reasoning become clouded. Sattvic is the purest diet, promoting a balanced flow of energy and calmness allowing the mind to tune-into meditation and concentration with more ease. These foods are vegetarian, nutritious, non-stimulating and non-irritating. *Mind is formed from the subtlest portion of the essence of food.* So if Sattvic is taken one step higher we have the Natural Hygiene and Living Foods. These are the tendencies I've noticed.

What are your thoughts about relationships? Many people just getting into a raw diet have problems because their mates don't want to change. Do you have any com-

ments or suggestions?
Truly, this can be a big challenge, especially if children are already in the picture. It's an issue not easily answered from the perspective of an outsider looking in. New options may have to be created if an amenable respect and understanding between both parties cannot be met. *Change your diet to vegetarian live food choices, change your body's internal balance...change your body's internal balance, change your perceptions...change your perceptions, change your world!* I feel one's choice of mate should reflect similar lifestyle growth or a shared desire for it. In my opinion, this type of harmony is essential if both are to continue to evolve spiritually with little conflict. If children become part of a future plan, they will have a superior start, as well.

Do you think it's harder for a woman to eat a raw diet than it is for a man?
I think it's an individual call...male or female.

Why do you think there are more raw men than raw women?
Nature Cure was developed in Germany around 1822. The advent of Naturopathy came on the scene in the early 1900's, and Natural Hygiene appeared about fifty years ago. With all due respect to the great accomplishments of those early pioneers and visionaries, they nonetheless lived in a very chauvinistic era and attracted a high percentage of male proponents. Since then, many people from all walks of life have gone through the various living food-oriented health centers, clinics, organizations, restaurants, support groups, websites, and events, educating themselves with various publications. This, coupled with the explosion of a youthful trend over recent years, ushered in large measure through Nature's First Law, makes me wonder if a survey should be taken to assess what the *true* ratio is today! But without a doubt, information regarding female health in relation

to the Natural Hygiene/Living Food Lifestyle is barely surfacing at this point in *her story*. The more women learn about how superior nutritional support and exercise can positively effect menstruation, pregnancy, the health and genetic vitality of a child, menopause, physical beauty, aging and emotional/spiritual balance, the more they will want to adopt these principles. So certainly, this deficit must be corrected and developed ASAP. Our happiness, strength, direction of future generations, and environmental health depend on it!

What are your thoughts about the female menstruation cycle?
I had the privilege of posing that question to several women who have been long-time living foodists. Each reported that the pain associated with menstruation was significantly reduced or eradicated. I was a few years into the transition, having accomplished over 25 juice cleansing days (accumulated over this time, not all at once) when I noticed pain had decreased and duration lessened. Years later and directly after my first Guided Hygienic Fast, the cycle manifested no pain and lasted for 2 to 3 days. Today I experience little to no discomfort and cycle duration is still 2 to 3 days. BUT if I choose to consume more cooked food within the course of one or two consecutive months, menstruation pain appears and the cycle can last an extra day.

Do you think it is natural for a woman not to bleed when she is on a raw diet?
If there is no blood, it may be a good idea to seek the advice of a Natural Hygiene Consultant who understands female cyclic activity and can give a more thorough analysis of one's *individual* criteria, just to be sure. I am not convinced that it is a completely normal condition, although some living food women have told me that it was fine for them.

Do you have any comments about pregnancy and the raw diet?
Giving the best to a growing fetus is what all good mothers strive to do. I had the rare privilege to learn from quite a few women who've brought through children in this way. They report that the body responds better to the dramatic changes of pregnancy. This all depends on many factors including how cleaned-out mom was before-hand. Furthermore, moms say that kids rarely, if at all, suffer from common infant through childhood maladies (ear infections, fevers), reflecting their alert, calm, even-tempered and content dispositions. On the flip-side, and part of an ideally wonderful scenario, the father-to-be who enjoyed a Living Food lifestyle which included fasting, could plant seeds imbued with greater genetic vitality and strengthened traits. The child gets a great start, as do generations to come! We don't need to create perfect humans from laboratory petri dishes. The perfection is right here within us, if we create the correct conditions and choices.

Thank you for giving this interview. Is there anything you would you like to add?
We are eternal spirits in this temporary physical experience. Spending time on spiritual-emotional growth, compassion in action, meditation and exercise, coupled with living food consumption are the true essentials. Clearing the mind through meditation is most significant. For the body will someday decompose but spirit continues. The body is a brilliant tool which, when given the correct fuel, is designed to help us reach our highest aspirations! May all humanity and life forms attain peace and happiness.

Thank you Paul for giving me this opportunity to share.

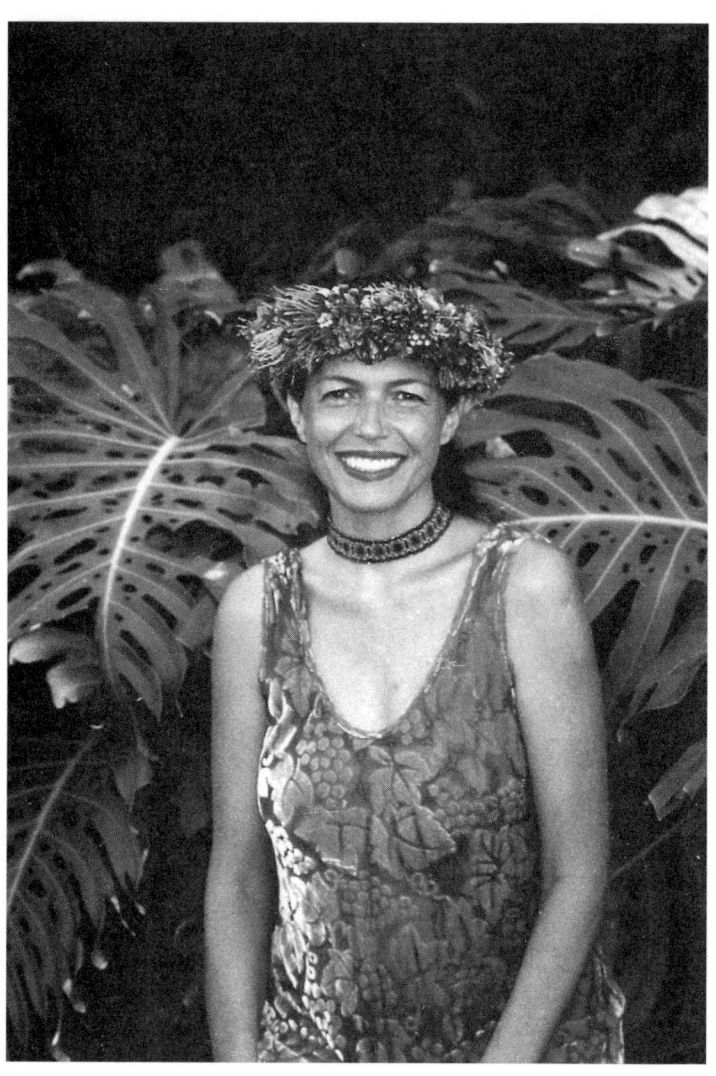

You may contact Katharine at:

800-927-2527 x 202
Email: HealthworksHI@aol.com

Katharine Clark

Katharine has held several positions in the health field over the years. At present, she is the CEO/President of Health Works Enterprises, Inc. and has built, and currently enjoys, a multi-million dollar network marketing company business with Cell Tech, organic whole food supplements.

Katharine was also a traveling holistic health consultant and trainer for many years in which she designed and delivered 3-day business and health training sessions, delivered in more than forty different cities per year in the United States and Canada, helping people basically understand their physiology holistically, the simple things that create a health promoting lifestyle and effect a measurable behavior modification.

She has also designed and conducted a one week residential retreat in Oregon for 60 to 80 women each year before the annual corporate conference. Retreat included educational classes and recreational activities. She created a team to continue producing the event when she retires from that job.

She also was a holistic health consultant and practitioner with extensive private practice experience extending from one on one counseling and evening educational courses, to private duty nursing for the seriously ill.

Katharine is also certified in: Alchemical Hypnotherapy, Reflexology, Colon Hydrotherapy, Iridology, Body Centered Psychoawareness, etc.

Educational background:
A.S. in Nursing, Indiana University, 1979
B.A. in Psychology, Indiana University, 1981
Certified Massage Therapist and Colon HydroTherapist, Florida School of Massage, 1982

Certified Iridologist, Rebirther, etc.

She has licenses in:
R.N. in Florida
L.M.T. in Florida

What are your height, age and weight?
I'm 5'6", forty-five and weigh 140 pounds.

When did you first start eating a raw food diet and what got you into it?
I got started twenty years ago in 1981 with raw living foods. My father was a butcher and I saw animals being slaughtered every single day. I wanted to be a vegetarian from the time I was a very young child. But, where I grew up in the Mid West, there weren't too many vegetarians. I was from a really small town, but I read most of the sacred teachings of the world. When I finally got away from Indiana, I used to look for anybody wearing Birkenstocks or girls who didn't shave their legs. I would go up to them and ask them if they were vegetarian, and eventually, I met some vegetarians. That was really wonderful. One girl in particular took me under her wing and we use to make tofu tuna sandwiches. That's what I remember the most. We became close buddies and I learned a lot from her. I ate the way she ate. I was using vegetarian cookbooks, but the foods were all cooked. I had no clear distinction about being vegan at all. Then I moved further south where there was a co-op health food store. It was in Cocoa Beach, Florida called the Sun Seed Co-op. The fellows running that co-op were living a vegan lifestyle.

One of them, Keith Peters, was vegan and also into raw foods. I went to him for reflexology. He started to share information with me about enzymes, raw foods and their benefits. Then I met two other fellows who were also into raw foods. They were all very helpful to me in my search for excellent health. I immediately became a raw foodist, becoming a vegan overnight on New Years Day, 1981.

I read books by Viktoras Kulvinskas, Morris Krok, Hilton Hotema and whatever else I could get my hands on at that point. I really wanted to feel good, have energy and be vibrantly alive. I wanted spiritual clarity, and I believed that eating live raw vegan food made the most sense. In 1983, I visited the Hippocrates Health Institute in Boston. At that point my partner and I had a non-profit "LifeMobile" which was a mobile alternative energy demonstration center and living foods kitchen. We could feed 250 people everyday with a salad topped with seed cheese and sauerkraut. It was a fun project and we ended up at the Miami Dade Community College in 1985 with a Home Self-Sufficiency Program in the Environmental Demonstration Center. It was a great opportunity and we had a regular program of 60 different classes a week.

Have you eaten 100% raw foods for all the years since you first tried it? If not why?
For the first eight years I was 100% raw vegan. Since then I have been 100% raw and other times, not. Now, I would say that I am more than 95% raw. Currently, I might eat some animal products, such as raw goat cheese. I occasionally use cooked sweeteners like Maple or Agave in my tea. If I'm in a situation where only cooked foods are available, I don't make a big deal of it – if someone invites me out for dinner. If there's a way to avoid it, I do.

I got away from eating 100% raw when I was traveling abroad and I would go into people's homes. They would take a week or a month of their resources to give me dinner. Before I learned how to avoid those situations, I felt as if I needed to say thank you and eat whatever was presented to me.

Also in 1991, my vegan physician told me that I needed to eat meat. I tried, and it did actually did improve my condition. Then over the years, I strayed more and more often until I just had to stop. My inner guidance tells me that raw is best! I think it was a good experience because I learned to forgive myself and to love myself more by eating raw. One learns from straying and learns to listen to how the body responds. These learning experiences can be valuable. Don't beat yourself up for them.

Can you talk about how eating live food has reached you on a spiritual level?
Sure. I certainly needed the change to live foods for my health because I had low energy and chronic depression to the point of suicidal thoughts. But the change to live foods was more a spiritual pursuit than something I thought was good for the environment or my health. I could feel the spirit guiding me to this path.

The raw food diet is spiritually enhancing. We talk about cleaning out our arteries, detoxifying and cleaning out our tissues, but we are also cleaning out our spiritual bodies. You are becoming more permeable, in cellular membranes, as well as in your spiritual body. As you eat more raw foods, you become more able to hear you own inner voice and your own inner guidance, which is very important. Spiritual realization is very important to me.

I kind of went through an adolescence on my path – straying, experimenting. I learned to love myself and not punish myself or wallow in guilt. That is why I've not been as rigid and dogmatic at maintaining the diet as I was at first, and why I've tried other things. To be in moderation means not being rigid or dogmatic.

For the first seven years, I never ever cheated. I never ate anything that wasn't raw food and vegan. I gained a lot from that. Afterwards, I was able to eat things that before would have sickened me. I got a whole lot healthier. I learned to love myself even when I wasn't eating my "righteous" diet.

After having been so rigid for seven years, what finally made you decide to eat some cooked food or even some animal products? What caused that to happen?
When I was in Bombay, I met a fellow who had studied with Rajshinesh. He had done quite a bit of spiritual practice and began teaching and training me. He had been a vegetarian and he said, "This is ridiculous, it's not about what you eat; you can eat anything." He encouraged me to eat something else, and I ate a lobster. I did not go completely off my path at that point, however that was an isolated incident. The interesting thing is, I did not get sick from eating that lobster. At that point I returned to mostly raw – but had some soups and greens in Thailand, mostly because of lack of availability of other things. In Nepal, I ate some Tibetan momos, which are like dim sum. When I was in Asia, I went into people's homes and saw the energy, the love with which they prepared food, and how important it was to them. They were giving so much to have me as a dinner guest. Even though sometimes the food was awful, I ate it with gratitude. I just thought, "How can I say 'no thank you' to these people."

My most significant diversion came in 1991 when my vegan doctor told me I needed to eat meat. This led to a whole expedition back into the SAD (Standard American Diet). Eventually, the exception became the rule. In early 2001, I was 80% raw, but ate lamb once a month. After attending the Portland Living Foods Festival in June, I rededicated myself to vegetarianism and eating raw and live food. I don't regret my straying because I learned from it. For one thing, from being raw for so long my digestion had very much improved, I could eat cooked food and still feel good. It was an affirmation of the healing power of eating live and raw.

As a woman, do you see any differences between men and woman eating this type of diet?
Everyone is different and finding one's own way is always an important individual pursuit. I think perhaps it can be more challenging for women, who experience emotional swings and cravings around their menstrual cycle, to stick with raw during that time. Being pregnant is also an emotional time and can lead to challenges. I recommend finding a support person or group, whether you're having challenges or not, to support you in your live food lifestyle changes.

Have you seen any connections with that at all?
About four years into being all-raw, I found myself craving chicken and I realized through interviewing myself that what I was hungry for was the Sunday afternoon dinner that I used to have with my family. When my parents and I sat down around the table on Sunday, we ate chicken from our farm. I realized that what I was hungry for was that feeling of love and being with my family and all those good feelings.

Regarding the menses, I've often said, "if a guy ever stood up from a toilet and saw it full of blood, he would freak out!" That's what happens to women! I mean it is freaky to have blood running out of you! It is scary, and of course you might be emotional about it. Then there are the physical changes, the hormonal changes which can make you emotional. That could definitely make it more difficult to stay on your diet at that time. When I first started out, I was so absolutely strict. Later, I realized that in a way, I was trying to eat my way to heaven. It was a way of being self-righteous because now I ate righteously. I was brought up in a Southern Baptist home and I became a missionary for raw foods, with the same kind of missionary zeal that colonized the planet in the past. Now, I don't feel that way. I don't feel that if a woman is raw, gets her period, and goes and eats something off her diet, that it's the end of the world. I don't get into the shame thing at all. If you stray, you can begin a new day and start all over again with a new resolve to eat light and feel bright! If you're an average person looking to improve your health or open your spirituality, I think it's better, to not beat yourself up over those things. Just get yourself back on the path.

Have you noticed any changes in your menstrual cycle from before you were eating raw until now?
I have not noticed a big difference. I have rarely had painful or long periods. When I was sixteen, I had no flow for over a year anyway. Youkta, my mentor, whose interview is also in this book, shares these experiences. I've learned from her that although she has had no monthly flow for years, if she eats something heavy in protein, then she will bleed. She still has sensations of her cycles. Eating chocolate is one major cause of difficult menstruation and PMS. Coffee is another offensive food that will cause difficulties with the cycle.

If there were a young girl making the change to a raw food lifestyle experiencing the phenomenon of having no blood flow during her menstrual cycle, would you think that it is healthy or natural?
I think not to bleed is a very healthy and natural occurrence. You can still have ovulation. You can still conceive when you are not having your period. I know many women in the raw food movement who do not bleed monthly and have been able to have children. Some of them have had several children, and they did not get their period back in between the births either. I've definitely seen woman whose difficult periods and heavy flows became lighter, and their period became a breeze once they followed a raw food diet. Most of the time, when I get my period, I have no signs that it's coming. It's pain-free.

What are some challenges not only for women, but also for all people in general making the change to a raw

food lifestyle?
First and foremost is the lack of understanding of friends, family and society at large. I get the "Oh, you can eat this, (pointing to a steak) right?" thing all the time. There are many more folks who are unsupportive rather than supportive of being raw or just vegetarian. Some may even be hostile or try to make you afraid. Some folks will laugh at you and make fun – simply out of ignorance, I might add. That's why reading books, getting to the website chats and finding a buddy or mentor is important.

Secondly, one must educate oneself. Eating only fruits leads to losing teeth! Eating sweets all the time, dried fruits and nuts, isn't healthy either. So, as one reads, learns, attends educational events and tries things out, it can be difficult. Also, some foods, like rolled oats, nori, cashews, are already cooked even when labeled raw. So one must study as well as experiment. www.living-foods.com is a good place to research for information and resources. I think it's important to find mentors, read books, listen to tapes, research the web. There are so many more resources available than when I was initially doing this.

I remember being so hungry and eating so many nuts that I made myself sick. I remember doing that liver flush thing and almost dying. Some of your lessons are going to be learned the hard way – through personal experiences. That's the way life is. I would warn against eating exclusively only a few different items. Going for a variety of foods will avoid pitfalls. You might eat just one thing at one meal, but you don't want to eat that one same thing for every meal.

Remember to drink plenty of water especially in the beginning. It's been said to drink half of your body weight in ounces every day. This is so important especially in the beginning to help elimination. Water is needed in every cell of the body and most people are chronically dehydrated. Of course, structured water from coconuts or watermelons is desirable.

Purified, filtered, reverse osmosis, ozonated water is preferable to spring water or distilled water. Later, eating higher water content foods may make drinking this much water unnecessary. When you have more experience you'll know.

I've found that using organic super foods like dried wild algae, grasses, sprouts and greens, food enzymes and probiotics makes the transition easier and brings the results you're looking for more quickly and consistently. If you have a serious health problem, eating super foods will be a huge benefit. I work with Viktoras Kulvinskas, and we highly recommend super foods. Adding them to your diet will help you avoid much of the discomfort of cleansing and the tendency to stray off the diet.

I think it's just good to be gentle with yourself, and just do the best you can as you continue to learn more and more. Getting into this lifestyle is about loving yourself. You are doing it to get healthier and to be more spiritually aware and to open up your own intuition. I really want to encourage people to be gentle with themselves as they would with an infant.

What about pitfalls concerning the issues of weight loss or weight gain for people new to a raw food diet? Any comments about that?
Most people do lose some weight when they begin an all raw diet, but after a while their weight will normalize. I actually got very thin initially. I do not have that weight problem now. If you are dangerously thin, then contact one of the leaders in the movement and get some help. Because if you go to a regular practitioner, like my practitioner who said, "You're going to have to eat meat, you're going to have to eat cooked food." This is what they might tell you because they haven't had an education on the benefits of living and raw food. But if you go to one of the leaders we now have in our field, who has been doing this for ten to thirty years, he or she will be able to help coach you through that.

Weight gain or loss can also be a result of emotional problems, just as it is for cooked food eaters.

Once you're all transitioned, you may find some foods more fattening. I have learned from my raw friend, that she will gain weight if she eats bananas or avocados. Some people will gain weight if they eat nuts, and other people won't.

Just do the best you can and you'll find your way.

How much weight did you lose once you started the raw food lifestyle, and how did you deal with the weight loss?
The interesting thing is that I lost about ten pounds when I started this program and I weighed 120 pounds. When I was younger, I had done a lot of drugs and I had weighed 120 pounds and everybody said I looked like death, but when I weighed 120 pounds after being on the raw food diet, everyone was saying, "Oh, you look fabulous!."

What is your opinion on exercise?
Exercise is vitally important, whether you walk, run, lift weights, swim, play tennis or row. If you don't have any kind of physical activity, no matter what you eat, you are not going to build your muscles and feel optimal.

Especially for raw fooders who have gotten really, really thin, or who have a tendency to be too thin, exercise is the key for them to build their body mass again. Working out in the gym, doing weight bearing kinds of exercise, will put weight back on them.

What do you think are the two most important things people should realize when considering making a change to a raw food lifestyle?
It may be hard in the beginning, but the benefits are going to more than outweigh any struggles. That is for sure. If you miss the tastes of certain foods at first, later on your tastes will change. You're going to see how fabulous foods can taste. Raw whole foods begin to taste so much better than cooked

foods ever did. You will definitely develop new food traditions, new comfort foods and new holiday foods.

You will settle into a program that feels very good, and easy for you to follow. Your appetites will change and eating raw will not be a struggle or a discipline. You won't even consider eating anything else. When you stray it's OK. Just get back with the program and realize that your experiences will be an inspiration to someone else someday who's having trouble straying too. You'll be able to say that you've had that experience too, but you made it through to the benefits of the live food lifestyle and so will they. Eventually even your family will admit your success.

How is your health and energy?
Currently, my energy is really fantastic. What I've noticed before I went on raw foods is that even though I was still in my twenties, I was still in a very degenerated, enzyme depleted condition. I did not have energy to do the things I wanted, and I was very depressed. Going on raw foods, I really felt like a child again. I felt I had the opportunity to experience things that I had never experienced before, even as a child: playing, being able to move freely in my body. It liberated my body, mind and spirit a great deal. I had a great deal more physical energy. I also needed a lot less sleep than before. I just think there is a vibrancy that comes to anyone emotionally, physically and spiritually when eating fresh, raw and organic foods. Earlier, I had mentioned having become more connected to my own inner guidance and my own inner voice. This makes me happy.

Out of all the foods out there, raw or cooked, what is your favorite?
Mangos! Mangos are my favorite. It's interesting because the doctor said they are good for rebuilding the adrenals. They are my favorite food. A couple of months ago, I had black

sapotes and they were my favorite food while they were available. Now, I'm eating black cherries and they've been a favorite since childhood. I also like hijiki. Oh, so many things are good. I'm not that fussy. I just like to eat!

Can you talk about the relationship between the raw food diet and environmental climate conditions?
Many people get cold easily after they start eating a living food diet. If they weren't cold natured before, they might even become cold natured. I often hear folks say, "Eating raw is OK for the tropics, but not if I live where it's cold." I started doing this in Florida. Then, I started living in Santa Fe, New Mexico. Santa Fe is a very, very cold place. Once again, I called on my mentor, Youkta, to help me, and she pointed out that some foods are warming and some foods are cooling. Vegetables such as beets and carrots, she said, were warming. We also ate sprouted grains when it was cold and they were very beneficial for women's hormonal systems. When you live where it's cold, it's even more important not to eat or drink cold foods. When it is cold outside, you might want to let your foods warm up to room temperature, or even make them with warm liquids. If you've made juice for yourself, you might want to make sure it warms up before you drink it.

Since you also want to drink your juice as soon as you can after you've made it, you can even warm it up a little. Of course, you only want to warm it up only to the point that it feels warm to your finger, and not end up cooking it. Those hints will help you stay warm in the colder climates. Once you're into this a while, your tissues will get cleansed and you'll have the improved circulation to stay warm.

Exercising will help too. What helped me the most to finally get my inner fire burning is the practice of QiGong. Now I can make myself hot without even moving by doing my practice.

Eating locally grown food is important. It's much more desirable than eating food that has been shipped into your area.

Getting local foods and eating them will help you adjust to the local climate. So, if you live where it's cold, you'll be eating nuts, seeds, ferments, dried fruits and vegetables, grasses, greens, sprouted pulses more than imported fruits.

In terms of relationships, mates or spouses, if one person is eating a raw food diet and the other is not, or if both have not and one person changes, what is your opinion on how to deal with that?
Being in a relationship with someone who is still eating cooked food certainly led me to eating more cooked food. Being in a relationship with someone who eats all raw was an education and inspiration for me and led me to eat more raw foods. I am a Pisces and have a tendency to go with the flow. In one of the significant relationships of my life, he wasn't raw, but I was able to teach him, and he was interested in feeling better. He was interested in the benefits. He took a great interest in it. So, in that case, I influenced him. I, personally, wouldn't want to be with someone who is eating meat and eating mostly cooked foods. I certainly wouldn't prepare cooked foods for him. So, I'd like my boyfriend to be into the raw living healthful, spiritually opening lifestyle as I am.

What is your opinion on how people can deal with their cooked food family members who will not listen?
It was difficult for me when immediate family members and loved ones got sick and kept eating the Standard American Diet. Their conditions could have improved had they changed their lifestyles and dining habits, but I watched my dad, mom and brother die. Who am I to say that they weren't fulfilling their highest life's purposes? I don't want them to judge my lifestyle, so I cannot sit in judgment of theirs, even if they're killing themselves slowly with food and/or thought poisoning. Last year, one of my nephews had two heart attacks at thirty-five. My father had so many heart attacks, until the med-

ical profession said they could not do anything more for him. I took him to my doctor who worked on him for three hours and the following week, he had no chest pain at night, whereas before, he normally had horrible chest pain all night. He had also lost eighteen pounds. He and my mother decided it was too far a drive for them to go back to my doctor. I realized that every person on the planet has his own path to follow. In the Bible, it's written: "It is up to each man to work out his own salvation." I don't know what their karma is. Maybe they do know what's best for them. I trust that they lived their lives perfectly. I continued to be an example. I talked with them, offered them food. I brought dishes to family meals, some of which they liked and asked for again and again. Before my brother died, I would go to his house for my birthday and he would get everything from the health food store and make a special meal for me. I really enjoyed this, and I feel the benefit outweighed the loss of eating cooked food. These meals created some of the best, closest family times I've ever enjoyed. They all knew that I was making an exception to be with them. I always brought the salad and a fresh fruit pie which they enjoyed with me. They even wanted the recipes sometimes!

I really changed, from the way I was at first, that is being very judgmental and absolutely never eating anything they ate. But as my mother aged, and it became obvious she wasn't going to live much longer, I had alternatives for her that I know would have kept her alive and made her more comfortable. But she wasn't at all interested. So, I spent time with her, and sometimes I would even eat cottage cheese and tomatoes with her because she had very little appetite and that's what she wanted to eat. I ate it just to be with her and not to be in a judgmental space with her. I ate it just to let her know that I loved her, and really appreciated her being my mother and everything she did for me. I showed her that I respected her and her choices, just as I wanted her to respect my choices. She hadn't laid trips on me and I realized I needed to stop laying trips on her. It might not be an option for you to ever eat cooked food under any circumstances and that's okay too. I don't think that means you can't love and be close to your family too. This is just how I went about it in the last few years when I had already become less strict with my own diet.

This summer, my niece, who is twenty-six, and her daughter who is seven, visited me in Hawaii. While they were there, they did not taste any of the foods we made. They did not want to taste pineapple or papaya. They would not taste the mangos. They would not drink the coconut water, not even a taste! One day, they went into the store at the gasoline station. They came out with their food. That's what they ate all week long: coke, pop tarts, whatever. I found it very interesting and actually kind of amusing, because I often joke about the food in those stores (or the lack of it). I wondered who could actually find any kind of food in one of those stores. Now, I know. Still, we had one of the best visits we could have had together. I didn't lay any trips on them, and they didn't lay any trips on me. I still made living raw foods available for them everyday and offered them at each opportunity, but I didn't ridicule their choices. Maybe next time they'll be more adventurous. They are well aware of my lifestyle without my preaching to them or acting as if they were crazy for killing themselves with their diets. I know my family can see that my lifestyle keeps me healthy.

For the holidays, I almost always send my family living foods recipe books with a note suggesting that everyone could benefit from eating more raw foods. Sometimes I send dehydrated fruit cookies or crackers, but I doubt they even eat them. They have their own lives. I'm not going to let my diet come between our love.

I am not an inclined to eat cooked food at this point,

though since my parents are gone. I can just as easily eat a salad without making a big deal of it. You'll know what to do with your family and friends. You can try it both ways and see what feels good to you.

Recently I was traveling for two months on the mainland. Everywhere I stayed with friends, I made living foods. For one meal, I made the spiral slicer angel hair from zucchini with fresh tomato sauce and macademia nut cheese. Everyone loved it! I should get a commission on those spiral slicers, I sold so many! I made fresh juices. I bought home fresh fruits. I didn't make a big deal of eating all raw or vegetarian. Everyday, I just contributed a little bit of fresh and raw food to the household. At one place they said, is it okay if we make steaks on the grill too? I said sure. They asked if I wanted steak too. I said no. It turned out they loved the spaghetti and several folks asked for the recipe so they could have it again. A couple of them asked for recipe books. I felt really good about it. After all, everyone knows that everyone stands to benefit from eating more living raw foods.

Where do you see the raw food movement in the future?
Today, almost everyone in America knows that they can benefit from eating more raw food. As more celebrities get into the live/raw foods diet, it will become even more popular. As people experience the benefits, it will remain part of their lives.

Economist Paul Zane Pilzer predicts a one trillion dollar wellness industry by the year 2010. He states, "Today, the food industry represents about one trillion dollars annually: the 'sickness business' (the current medical system) is another trillion. These two industries feed one another in a fairly insidious way because such a huge part of sickness today is caused by the poor nutrition supplied by the food industry." He defines "wellness" as money spent to make you feel healthier, even when you're not "sick" by any standard medical terms. He predicts that the "39% of Americans who are not overweight comprising 10 - 15 million people, as they age, are getting healthier, more fit, stronger - actually younger, by any standard medical definition. These people represent that new economic sector. The first thing they do, as they start to have money, is to figure out how they can be healthier - and they're doing it outside the medical establishment. In the year 2000, wellness in America was already a 200 billion dollar industry. Baby Boomers are the first generation we know of in recorded history who refuse to accept the aging process." (Quotes from Network Marketing Lifestyles Vol. 3, Issue 5, Interview with Paul Zane Pilzer).

Of course we know that eating live/raw will retard the aging process, so it's just a matter of time before this is big - very big.

Would you like to add anything else before we end this interview?
I would encourage you to make a commitment to eating live and raw food. Do your best to stick to it. Keep a diary of your gains and successes and experiences. Encourage those around you to eat more fresh, raw and vegan. Enjoy the benefits!

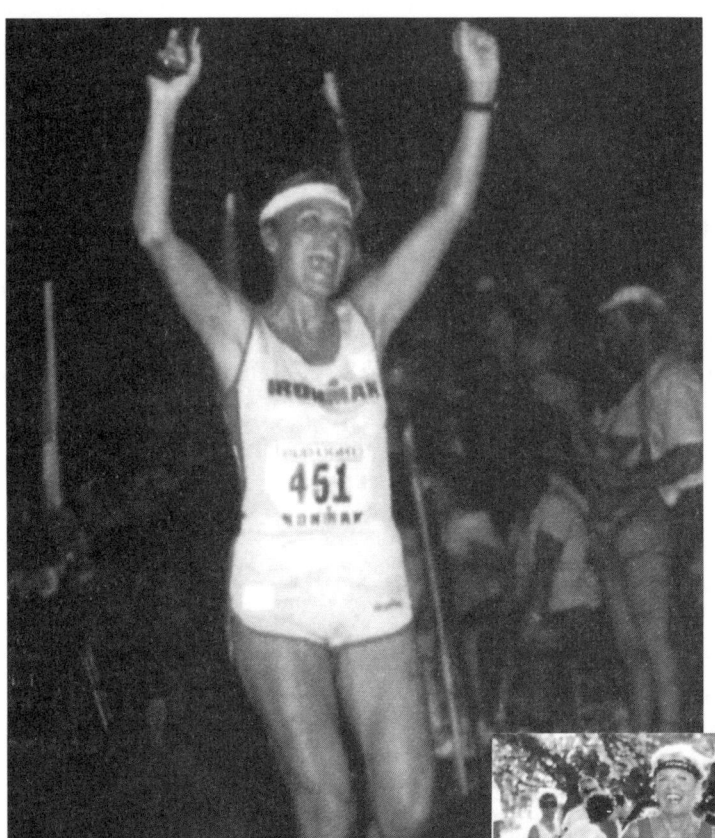

You may contact Ruth at:

Ruth E. Heidrich, Ph.D.
1415 Victoria St. #1106
Honolulu, HI 96822

Ask Dr. Ruth: vegsource.com
Website: http://www.ironlady.com

Ruth Heidrich

Dr. Ruth Heidrich holds a B.A. and a Master's Degree in Psychology, and earned a Ph.D. in Health Management in 1993. She is the author of *A Race For Life* and *The Race For Life Cookbook*.

She is a certified fitness trainer and has held three world records for fitness for her age group at the renowned Cooper Clinic in Dallas, Texas. She still actively competes in marathons and triathlons and has won more than 800 trophies and medals since her diagnosis of breast cancer in 1982 at the age of 47.

With Terry Shintani, M.D., she has co-hosted the radio show *Nutrition and You* on KWAI-AM in Hawaii for 14 years.

Ruth is past president of the Vegetarian Society of Hawaii and the Mid Pacific Road Runners Club. She won four gold medals in the 1997 Senior Olympics, held in Las Vegas, Nevada.

Ruth is an internationally acclaimed author and lecturer, speaking at conferences around the world.

At the age of 63 in 1997, Ruth completed 63 races - triathlons, biathlons, runs, and bike races. She was aiming for 64 races for her 64th year, and by April 22, 1998, she had already won 20 additional races, including two on the previous weekend. "I wanted to show that it is possible to grow stronger as you grow older," she says. "I was going to be proof that you could."

Then, while on a bike training ride, a truck driver coming in the opposite direction, suddenly saw the street he was looking for, turned and slammed right into her. "You know how they say that your life flashes before you just before you die?" Ruth asks. "As I was flying through the air, the future flashed before my eyes. I knew that my goal of competing in all these races was about to be over. And at that point, I was in the best physical condition of my life. The injuries turned out to be worse than I could possibly imagine. Both my left leg and right hip had sustained multiple fractures." In the Emergency Room, the doctors, when assessing the damage, said that if she hadn't been in such good physical condition, she probably would have been killed, the impact was that hard.

She began physical therapy within two weeks, but progress came slowly. "The worst day," she says, "was about three months later when the doctor said that I needed to accept that I would never run again, much less race." In response, she doubled her physical therapy. Since her health plan only covered two days per week, she added two more days and paid for them herself.

Today, Ruth is back competing again. She says with a laugh, "I've got all these doctors shaking their heads." She recently completed the Hickam and the AARP Triathlons that were within a week of each other!

This wasn't the first time she had to bounce back. In 1982, she was diagnosed with breast cancer. "It was such a shock - as a 14-year-runner and marathoner, I was the healthiest person I knew," Ruth says. "But I kept on training, knowing the many benefits of running, including relieving stress. One of the doctors warned me to stop, saying, 'Lady, forget it; you're a cancer patient; you need to rest, to take it easy.'" Then, just two weeks after the cancer diagnosis, she saw an event on TV that was about to change her life: the Ironman Triathlon! This involved a 2.4-mile swim, followed by a 112-mile bike leg, and then a 26.2-mile marathon. With a sly chuckle, she decided to add biking and swimming to an already heavy running schedule. She found the more she did, the better she felt, and in 1984 she completed her first Ironman Triathlon! In 1986 she was invited to compete in both the New Zealand and Japan Ironman Triathlons, winning age-group firsts and setting national records in both.

At the same time she started training for the Ironman, she

investigated the role of diet in breast cancer and the research being conducted by Dr. John McDougall. "I enrolled in his clinical research study that required a vegan (strict vegetarian), low-fat diet," she says. "My cholesterol went from 236 to 160 in just 21 days. It later went down to 127 and eventually even lower. There were a lot of other benefits, too. I was running faster and enjoying it more." She also beat the cancer, it seems. "It led to my philosophy: You can do just about anything you want."

How many years have you been on the raw diet, and what got you into it?
I started the raw diet in 1998, mostly because of my speaking and racing schedule, which involves heavy travel. When you pull into a new town, you never know where to get good, healthy food. I'd been presented with that problem not only in this country, but also in Japan, Russia, New Zealand, China, etc. I never had cooking facilities, but I could always find a little food market or green grocer, so I did what was natural: buying fruits and vegetables and taking them back to my room and eating them!

How was your health when you started the diet?
I have to say that my health was pretty good in 1998, primarily because I was already following a vegan diet and had been for almost eighteen years. But when I went raw, I felt even better!

Who are some of the people who have inspired you to do this?
Dr. Bill Harris and Doug Graham helped by assuring me that I was better off without grains.

Is there any one person who has inspired you the most?
Actually, no, because the reason I did it was primarily the convenience and ease of eating this way. It's just so darned easy!

You've learned so much over the years. What are some of the most important things you've learned?
One of the most important things I've learned over the years is that plants are the proper fuel for the human body. Animals as food not only clog up the circulatory system and suppress the immune system, they are responsible for most of the diseases humans are subject to.

Are there any pitfalls that you have learned to watch out for on the raw diet?
I can't think of any!

Weight loss is a big pitfall for many people. Do you have any thoughts about that?
Weight loss is a misleading concept. We need to think in terms of "fat loss." When switching to raw, most people lose a lot of fat. If you are exercising vigorously on a daily basis, your muscles get stronger, so although the scales may or may not show a loss of weight, you are actually preserving muscle mass and lowering your body fat percentage.

Dental problems are another big pitfall. Any thoughts?
I don't know of any dental problems associated with going raw. I DO know that every time I go to my dentist for a check-up, she looks in my mouth, straightens up, and says to her dental assistant, "Now, THERE'S a healthy mouth! Just look at those beautiful teeth and gums! I wish all my patients looked like this!"

What are your thoughts about mercury fillings, and what would you replace them with?
I'm not an expert in this field, but both my dentist and I felt that I was better off without mercury, so we replaced my old fillings with porcelain.

What is your opinion of nuts and seeds?
I eat them only rarely because of their high fat and high pro-

tein content and the risk of their being rancid.

What is your opinion of grains?
I gave them up primarily because they are deficient in so many nutrients and inconvenient to prepare.

What is your opinion of sprouts?
I keep a "garden" in my kitchen with a continuous supply of mung bean sprouts by my sink.

What is your opinion of Natural Hygiene?
They are leaders in the health movement.

What is your opinion of supplements?
They provide nothing that I need that I can't get in fruits and vegetables.

What is your opinion of eating seasonally?
I prefer fruits and vegetables right out of the garden, but since that's rarely possible, I do the next best thing: shop in the produce section and buy what appeals to me.

What is your opinion of fasting?
I have not found it to be necessary, and the few times I tried it, I couldn't keep up my triathlon training schedule.

What is your opinion of food combining on a 100% raw diet, and is it necessary?
If it's necessary, I haven't found the reason. I just mix up fruits and vegetables any way that looks appealing.

What is your opinion of physical exercise?
Ha! I LOVE it. I run, bike, swim, and lift weights almost every day, and I frequently have trouble backing off. For example, you're supposed to "taper" before a major athletic event, and I say to myself the day before, "I'll just go for a short, easy run," but then I find myself saying, "Just one more mile and THEN I'll quit!" Most other athletes I know don't have trouble with tapering.

What is your opinion of wild foods?
I love to go on hikes and discover berries. Also, in Hawaii, there are lots of guavas and mangos just falling off trees. I load up my backpack and feast for days on my found treasures.

What are your age, height, and weight? Has your weight changed, or were there other changes your body went through? How did you handle it?
I'm now 67, about five feet eight inches tall (I've lost NO height as most people do by this age), and weigh about 125 pounds. My body fat percentage is 14 % (the average college-age female's is 30 %), and people frequently guess that I'm in my forties.

Since I started serious running in 1968, I have never had a weight problem. I have been extremely fit for over thirty years, but I was just not healthy! The diagnosis of breast cancer in 1982 shocked me and told me that I was not doing enough. That was the motivation to go vegan. That, of course, was a major step towards glowing, good health. The final step to raw came about primarily for convenience. It's so natural and makes so much sense that now I can't imagine eating any other way.

Did you ever get really sick or have a really bad detox?
No, not at all. I just started immediately feeling lighter, cleaner and faster.

Do you eat 100% raw foods, and if so, for how long? If not, why do you eat cooked foods, and what do you eat that is cooked?
The only deviation from 100% raw is as follows: small amounts of miso, blackstrap molasses, and nutritional yeast with B-12. If I were convinced that these are not good for me, I could easily give them up.

What is your average daily diet like? What do you eat

and how often?
I "graze," which means I have no special meal times. In general, my first meal of the day comes after a two-hour workout and consists of greens, a carrot, a banana, and a mango all cut up and blackstrap molasses, and nutritional yeast added and the whole thing mixed up. I've been eating this breakfast for years now and find that it is easy and satisfying and gets me ready for the rest of the day. I usually get hungry every two to three hours, so I will snack on carrots, greens, tomatoes, apples, cabbage, and dried fruit such as prunes and cranberries. These ingredients also make up my lunch and dinner with the addition of thinly sliced fresh raw ginger. I also love raw corn on the cob. For dessert, I eat berries of all kinds.

What is your favorite food?
Fruits of all kinds.

Out of all of the foods, what do you think is the most important?
Greens are extremely important, I think, because of their highest level of nutrient-per-calorie ratio.

How are your health and energy?
Fantastic! I've done events such as three marathons in three weeks and a total of 67 marathons. I've raced thirty-seven miles to the top of Haleakala on Maui, from sea level to 10,000 feet in seven hours and won an age-group First Place trophy. I've done an Ironman Triathlon one week and set a new State Record in the 25K race the next week. I've won more than 800 First Place trophies in races consisting of triathlons, road running, biathlons, pentathlons (I hold the State record in that one), and much more. I love racing.

How much sleep do you get, and how much do you think is necessary?
I usually get about five to six hours sleep a night. I get to bed

around midnight, and I'm up by 5:00 or 6:00 a.m., raring to go.

Have you noticed any mental changes?
Ah, much clearer thinking, greater awareness of my environment, and total empathy for animals, especially the ones most people call "food."

Many people just getting into a raw diet have problems because their mates don't want to change. Do you have any comments or suggestions on this?
Yes, that can be a major problem. Education is the key, as well as a willingness on the part of the other person to "just try it." I've converted lots of people in my time through this approach.

Do you think it's harder for a woman to eat a raw diet than it is for a man?
No, I don't see why it would be harder for a woman.

What are your thoughts about the female menstruation cycle?
I think the raw diet will help with the hormone balance and relieve many of the symptoms that women have, such as PMS, fibrocystic breasts, heavy bleeding, and menopausal symptoms.

Do you think it's natural for a woman not to bleed when she is on a raw diet, or should there be blood?
Since the bleeding is the shedding of the old endometrium, there will probably always be some bleeding, but not nearly to the extent that most women in Western societies experience.

Estrogen levels in women (as well as men) rise with the consumption of animal foods, and this causes over stimulation of the reproductive tissues of the body (breasts and uterus), which, of course, leads to cancer and other problems. This is compounded by the low-fiber (actually, NO-fiber) intake that comes with animal foods, which allows the estrogen to be re-absorbed into the bloodstream, thus compounding the problem.

Any comments about PMS and the raw diet?
PMS would probably totally disappear with a change to a raw diet.

Any comments about pregnancy and the raw diet?
I think intrinsically, a raw diet has got to be the best during pregnancy, but I can't really cite any research in this area.

Do you think it is easier to eat a raw diet today than it was years ago?
Yes, it's probably easier, mostly because there are a few more people leading the way.

Where do you see the raw diet in the future? Do you think it will ever go mainstream?
I think we have no choice but to go raw in the future. We certainly can't keep on doing what we're doing, for many reasons. We can't afford the health care costs, there soon won't be any more rain forests to cut down to graze cattle, and our rivers, streams, and oceans will get so polluted that we won't have any clean water to drink. I just did some talks and a race in Tulsa, Oklahoma, and one of the first things my host gave me upon arrival was a jug of distilled water. I looked a little surprised, so he explained that I would need this because the chicken farms upstream cause their water to stink!

Thank you for this interview. Is there anything else you would you like to add?
We humans have often gone down the wrong path. So far, we have been able to recognize it, back up, and change direction to the right path. This is where we are now. The scientific evidence is very clear that most of our diseases are diet-related and reversible by changing our diet. The planet is also in big trouble which, again, can be reversed by giving it a chance to revive; and of course, we need to realize that we are not the only creatures on this planet that have a right to live peacefully.

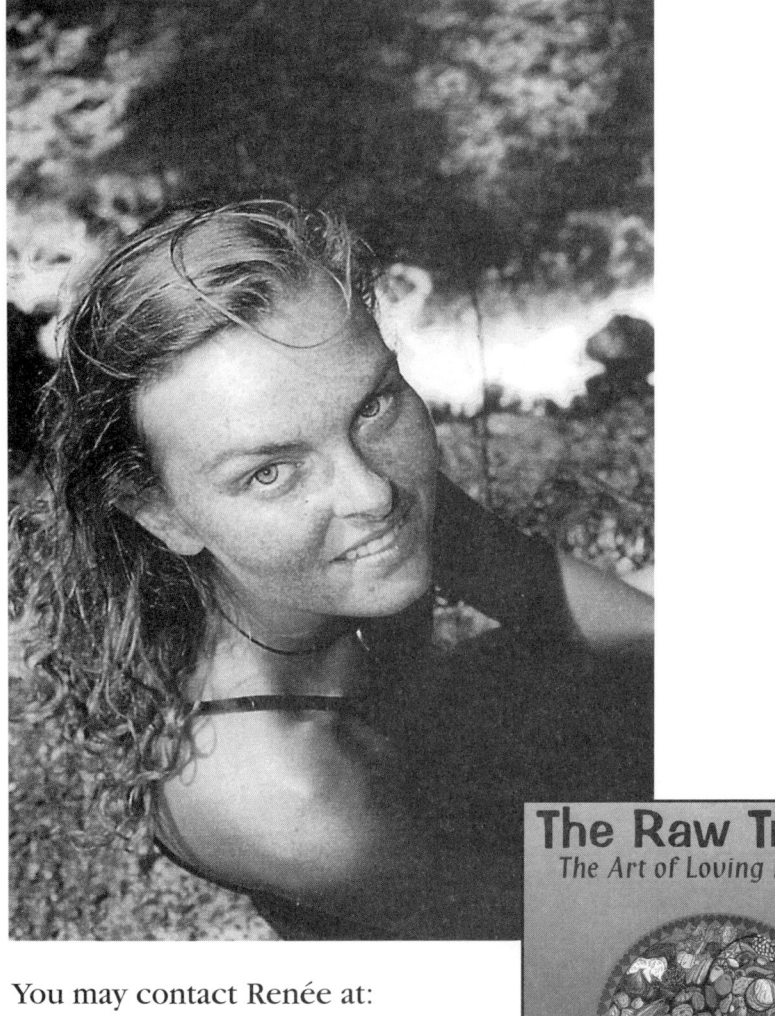

You may contact Renée at:

Renée Loux Underkoffler
Euphoric Organics
P.O. Box 790659
Paia Maui, Hawaii 96779
808-283-1833

E-mail: Reneeoflife@hotmail.com

Renée Loux Underkoffler

Renée is co-author of an excellent recipe book entitled *The Raw Truth: The Art of Loving Foods*.

Renée Loux Underkoffler is a renowned proponent and example of the Live-Foods lifestyle. She is a celebrated chef and dedicates her focus and talents to health and live-foods, nutritional education and the culinary arts of living foods.

Renée lives on the island of Maui, Hawaii for much of the year and teaches all over the world. She works privately in health counseling, cleansing and rejuvenation, and facilitates health retreats and workshops incorporating yoga, living-foods and balanced lifestyle. Institutions and corporations have welcomed her approachable healthful programs and insights into healthy living. Her successful focus aims at personal education and empowerment at the grass roots level and on red velvet carpets alike.

Renée co-founded *The Raw Experience Restaurant* in Paia, Maui in 1996. Her articles were published by many media interests for her delightful healthy living and sumptuous culinary creations. *The Raw Experience* featured the high ideals and discriminating standards of an organic, vegan, raw and living-foods menu supported almost exclusively by local, organic island farms. She taught a curriculum of culinary and live-food nutrition classes every week and provided a well-received nexus for education, gathering and a fabulous place to eat with live music on the weekends.

Renée co-published and illustrated *The Raw Truth: The Art of Loving Foods*, now in its fourth printing. An excellent guide to food, sprouting, and other information, *The Raw Truth* offers very approachable access to scrumptious raw and living foods recipes. She wrote a second recipe book, *Eu-*

phoric Organics, and a volume in progress, *The Science of Spiritual Nutrition: Seeds for Change*, a guide to comprehensive living nutrition and fine gourmet food, is due in the coming year.

One of Renée's feature projects this year was her involvement as a core member of the SOL tour (Simple Organic Living), a 1500 mile bicycle tour from Seattle, Washington to Los Angeles, with Woody Harrelson and a few friends, with speaking stops at nine universities. Followed by a tour bus called The Mothership which is decked on the inside with organic cotton and hemp and renewable cork and bamboo and runs on Biodiesel vegetable oil, they peddled from fifty to seventy miles a day, eating all organic raw foods that Renée prepared for the tribe in the bus kitchen, powered by solar panels. Several phenomenal keynote speakers including John Robbins, Howard Lyman and Julia Butterfly-Hill joined them as they presented their program to universities along the way between flurries of peddling. Thousands of students flocked to each venue: University of Washington, University of Oregon, Humboldt State, Sacramento State, San Francisco State, Stanford, Cal PolyTech, and University of Santa Barbara. There was incredible media coverage, and the stir was sensational. Each speaker talked about diverse aspects of Simple Organic Living and "leaving a light footprint" for a sustainable future. Renée spoke to the students about diet, sustainable agriculture and living foods for a living planet.

With the blessing and burden of a full film crew through every glorious and treacherous mile and venue, Ron Mann is producing a feature film about this adventure due to premiere in 2002.

Renée has been an inspiration and example of the live-foods lifestyle for more than seven years. She has a profound yoga practice and nurturing approach for whole health. Through experience and compassion, tailored to personal needs and challenges, she teaches people how to approach health and well being.

How many years have you been on the raw diet, and what got you into it?
The first cognitive thought I recall at the age of five was, "I will be a vegetarian when I turn eighteen." Age eighteen signified adulthood to my young years; I was at a loss to know that I could make qualified decisions at any age. I deeply loved animals and the outdoors. I realized that eating meat meant eating the flesh of a living creature. By the age of thirteen, I proudly declared my compassionate peace of mind and became a vegetarian.

By the time I attended University, I was well aware of the importance of organically grown food, wheatgrass, and fresh juices. I was a strict vegan, as were most of my near and dear friends. We preached like you can imagine. It was then that I learned that just being vegan does not mean being healthy. It is possible to be "vegan" and eat rubbish and an unbalanced diet. Then I began to learn about raw food and Yoga. I began to recognize that a combination of fresh, organic, raw food, yoga and exercise is a gorgeous formula for the body.

I had an epiphany during a bout of lung-and-tonsil infection that was caused by the artificial heat and air during the long East Coast winters. On a road trip to see The Grateful Dead with two great sisters, I was recovering from a bad cough. We were poor, and we drove a hovelled Oldsmobile. I was distraught, since we had no camping stove. My friend Sarah confidently told me that we would just eat all raw food. I exclaimed, "I can't eat all raw food; I am sick!" The moment she turned to me with bright green eyes and her pixie smile and said, "That is WHY we will eat all raw food," my life changed. The heavens opened. I got it.

Just about then, I met Jeremy Safron, who turned me on to a book that embodied my wildest dreams, titled *Survival into the 21st Century*, by Viktoras Kulvinskas. My eyes were opened. I realized that there was a movement and a science behind what I intuitively knew. I was no longer a freak waving my flag with uncertainty. I was hungry for knowledge. I read every book I could get my hands on and started whipping up wild concoctions. My yoga was blossoming and my mind blooming.

How was your health when you started the diet?
I have been active and athletic for the whole of my life. I did not come to Living Food because I was sick. I came to find how opulent health could be.

Who are some people who have inspired you to do this?
My inspiration was undoubtedly the grace and beauty of my longhaired mother, a pioneering vegetarian for most of her own years. A woman I met in college whose name I can't remember and Jeremy Safron have been invaluable partisans. The elders of the raw food movement have also inspired me to carry on the work: Dr. Ann Wigmore, Viktoras Kulvinskas, Dr. Gabriel Cousens, Herbert Shelton, and Paul Bragg, to name a few.

You've learned so much over the years. What are a few of the most important things you've learned?
The most important approach to true health and longevity is to be gentle and love ourselves. Diet is far more than what goes into our mouths. Peace of mind is the most profound and pervasive medicine. Loving your body is the most fundamental foundation for health. Attitude and intention are potent food for thought. Thoughts are potentially as toxic as any subject. Visualization is a powerful tool. What we focus on grows stronger. Love breeds life, health and balance. Homeostasis is maintaining a dynamic equilibrium in an ever-changing environment. This is the difficult task of balance in the body. There is an incomprehensible number of actions and reactions in our bodies every second. It requires the cooperation of every cell of every tissue, organ, gland, blood, and

bone to unify optimum life. Couple this process with the reality that we are constantly inundated with the ways of the world and the onslaught of physical influence. It's what I consider a moving MIRACLE. Our environment is continuously changing. Seasons, geography, emotional states, exercise, mental exertion, rest, and diet change are among many variables that significantly affect and influence our state of health. Maintaining balance is a full-time task for the body. Regular exercise is a key to keeping rhythm in the body. Yoga, deep breathing and stretching and strengthening the muscles is a formula for a happy mind and an ecstatic body.

Finally, committing to a personally realistic program will ensure lifetime success. It takes a mature and responsible honesty to recognize changing needs. Aspiring high and setting attainable goals is a measure for success.

Are there any pitfalls that you have learned to watch out for on the raw diet?
Dogma. "What doesn't bend, breaks..." I have seen people compromise their health in the name of preconceived beliefs that do not allow enough flexibility. Too much of anything is still too much. "Too much, too quick" is a recipe for chaos and disaster.

I often speak about homeostasis, which is maintaining a dynamic balance in a constantly changing environment. The influences on our body are many. Constant change calls for a sensitivity to changing needs. I have seen stubborn ways become a burden to health.
The end of the means is to respect our bodies, not any set of laws that we adhere to. Being gentle and accepting change lets everyone win.

Losing too much weight is a big pitfall for many people new to a raw food diet. Do you have any thoughts about that?

A common pattern on a completely raw food diet is an initial loss of weight followed by a regaining of balance. It can be determined that the body sheds tissue that has been built by a poor diet. With a good exercise program, new, healthy tissue will readily build. Exercise is also necessary for good weight balance. There is a formula to building and burning. I feel like I'm a good example of a strong woman with athletic endurance. I've been what I consider underweight during a time when I abstained from all oils including nuts and seeds. It was a good cleansing period, but not a recipe for the long run. With plenty of yoga and care, I found balance.

Dental problems are another big pitfall. Any thoughts?
Citrus and acidic fruit seem to be a culprit. Too much fruit in general seems to be a culprit. Yes, it is natural sugar, but sugar is sugar and it breaks down teeth. I take my oral hygiene seriously. Teeth brushing, tongue scraping, and flossing are essential. Brushing teeth after a meal is a good plan for prevention. What we brush our teeth with is just as important. Sodium-Laurel-Sulfate is detrimental to the system, especially the gums. Almost all toothpaste contains SLS. Weleda makes toothpaste without SLS. Weleda's "Sea Salt & Baking Soda" and "Plant Gel" are excellent. Sea salt and baking soda are good materials to whiten, but they should not be used too often because they are very abrasive. I rotate the two for balance. I use a Sonicare electric toothbrush in the morning and a regular brush at night. The Sonicare vibrates incredibly fast and massages the gums very well. Gum health = teeth health. It is a trade-off to use an electric machine in my mouth, but it is very effective. Tongue scraping is done with a curved metal instrument, easily obtained from a health-food store. It is estimated that 70% of the bacteria in your mouth is on your tongue. I scrape my tongue every time I brush. It helps keep the breath fresher than you might think. The edge of a spoon will work if you cannot find a scraper immediately. Flossing is

necessary to get into spots a brush cannot reach. It really is worthwhile to try and floss once a day. It is an effort, but I know I want my teeth for the rest of my life. Very diluted food grade Hydrogen Peroxide with tea tree oil is an excellent mouthwash to follow up with, scooting out all bacteria and yuckie from in between your teeth. The more your mouth foams and froths after you spit it out, the more work it is doing.

I have seen my teeth whiten and get strong from regularly swishing wheatgrass around in my mouth and chewing on the grass itself. I chew on licorice root regularly.

Chewing will strengthen teeth. Animals clean their teeth by chewing on sticks. Licorice will help whiten teeth as well as balance blood sugar and strengthen and balance the kidneys. Licorice is sweet tasting, and it's a good way to give the molars a workout. I give my teeth a lot of attention because I want to unabashedly smile my whole life. Cheers!

What is you opinion of mercury fillings, and what would you replace them with?
Undoubtedly, mercury is a dangerous poison that leaks into the body. There is a plethora of supportive information to avoid metals in the body, especially mercury. Unfortunately, I still have a bit of mercury-amalgam fillings wedged in my teeth.

Care certainly needs to be taken when removing mercury from the mouth. I have seen the detriments of poorly replaced cavities. There is a chance to further poison the body and wreck the mouth if fillings are not cared for with expert caution and skill. Metal poisoning is complexly hazardous. It is very expensive to seek out a qualified dentist to do the work, but it is unquestionably worth it. It is not worthwhile to risk hurting yourself through shoddy work.

There are several materials available to replace mercury. Gold is very pure and clean, although expensive. Porcelain looks nice since it is white, although it has been known to crack and it also must be shaped to perfection to fit the cavity. There are very hard plastic compilations that are reportedly excellent. Although it is plastic, a material we could do without in our bodies, it is apparently hard enough that there is little to no chance of any off-gassing or leeching into the body. Technology really seems to be in our favor on this one.

I recommend personal research into materials and a qualified dentist with references. You are worth the best.

What is your opinion of nuts and seeds?
Nuts and seeds are very concentrated nutrition. The protein and density are welcomed by many. They are most easily digested after soaking and made even more digestible by fermenting. The oils of nuts and seeds are very valuable. My favorite is the hemp seed out of its shell. Flax seed, chia seed, and pumpkin seeds are also high on my list. They have the best nutritional and essential fatty acid portfolio. I eat seeds and nuts quite sparingly, but I loyally rely on them for strenuous, high endurance adventures.

What is your opinion of grains?
I do not eat grains. There are so many options that are more digestible and have a better nutritional portfolio. The closest I come to eating grains is sprouted long-grain wild rice, which botanically is actually a seed.

What is your opinion of sprouts?
Sprouts are a super food. Sunflower, buckwheat, and clover are my favorites. Sprouts are a way to ensure fresh, local and organically grown food year-round in any climate.

What is your opinion of eating seasonally?
A seasonal diet makes perfect sense. It is a way for your body to calibrate to the environment. Eating locally grown produce is a socially, economically, and environmentally responsible choice. You benefit, the farmer benefits, and chances are that

little shipping and consumption of resources were involved in getting the food to you.

What is your opinion of fasting?
Fasting is undeniably a profound practice for regaining and improving health.

It is essential to fast responsibly and sensitively. There are many programs that have been successful and effective for many people. I personally endorse the Ejuva Cleanse with integrity. The herbs are all organic and wild, crafted from all over the world. The combinations are very effective and safe. I have worked with a broad spectrum of clients with this product with excellent results.

Herbs and programs can accelerate the healing process incredibly. Resting and refueling is one of the most considerable aspects of fasting. Breaking the fast gently and responsibly is the most important.

What is your opinion of exercise?
Yoga has been my personal practice for nearly a decade. It is part of my foundation. I practice at least an hour a day, no matter what. I practice first thing in the morning. It's a time I reserve to dedicate to my health, my body, and my mental and spiritual advancement. Yoga engages my body, mind and spirit in glorious union. Yoga is a practice for longevity. Far-reaching sight is essential for health. Healthy sutras that will carry the whole of our lives will grant a sense of grounding, regardless of the perpetual fluctuations of life.

What are your age, height, and weight? Has your weight changed, or are there any other changes your body has gone through? How did you handle it?
I am 26, five feet nine inches tall, and 130 pounds. For some time, I maintained an extremely strict diet. I did not eat any oil or nuts and very few seeds. I did not eat any grains or dehydrated food. I did not eat any refined food such as shoyu or

Bragg's. I fasted at least one day a week with longer fasts several times a year even when I was too busy to rest. I was extremely active, practicing yoga, kung-fu, running, and hiking. During that time, I lost quite a bit of weight. I felt well, though a little too thin. I required much less sleep, and I would wake before 6:00 a.m. every day. Certain aspects of such pious living were ideal in my life, but other considerations were lacking. For example, I bruised easily. Being so thin was great for yoga, but it left me feeling vulnerable and tired at times. I was quite socially retarded because I was so strict. Even when I made fantastic raw food meals, I made separate food for myself. I was at peace, but I could see friends and family growing uncomfortable.

I introduced flax and hemp oil into my diet and immediately felt a subtle satiation. My skin felt more hydrated and soft. I began to eat nuts and seeds and fasted less, and I was able to build more strength and endurance. I have evened out, and now I feel wonderful. I still fast several times a year, though more responsibly. I look like a vibrant, healthy woman. I feel strong and flexible in body and mind.

Do you eat 100% raw foods, and if so, for how long? If not, how much cooked food do you eat, and why?
I do not claim to be 100% anything but human. I do say that I live on a raw and live food diet. There are so many gray areas concerning what is considered raw and live. Miso, for instance, is a living food, but it is not raw. Nutritional yeast sits on the fence. Supplements vary. Even dehydrated food is frowned upon by some. I do drink tea. It has been a ritual for most of my life. I will put organic packaged almond, rice, or soy milk in it if I please when there is no fresh almond milk available.

Occasionally, I eat broccoli or asparagus that is lightly steamed because it is much more agreeable and digestible for my body, although, if I have time, I marinate it in the dehydrator long enough to achieve the same effect.

It does not seem worth the time or energy to bicker among ourselves about the details of marginal differences. I hope that all of us in the raw and live food movement will get together and agree that fresh, organic food is good for the body - the more the better. Concentrating on the good things we do for our bodies is much more fun than picking apart the rest.

What is your average daily diet like? What do you eat, and how often?

I eat very simply. I love to make decadent, gourmet food and serve it to loved ones rather than eat it.

I do not consume anything before yoga besides tea. I prefer to drink juice or eat fruit until noon. I drink wheatgrass and green juice every day that I can. I graze often, munching fruit and juices and lots of spirulina. I eat one main meal of the day. I generally prefer to eat mostly before sundown and lightly thereafter.

What is your favorite food?

I would say I like fresh green coconut water the best. I also love watermelon with seeds and spirulina flakes, as well as seaweed, and I love young, tender spinach.

Of all foods, which one do you think is the most important?

Enough greens for protein-building amino acids and macronutrients, good oil with essential fatty acids such as hemp and flax, and mineral-rich foods such as seaweed.

How are your health and energy?

I feel vibrant and full of energy. I am very physically active and mentally engaged. My skin is healthy, my eyes are clear, my teeth are white, my hair is soft and healthy, and all of the moons on my fingernails are well formed. I practice yoga, I meditate, I practice kung-fu and tai-chi. I run, walk, hike and bike. I read and study constantly. I write, do research and mentally challenge myself. I feel healthy and strong in body, mind, and spirit.

How much sleep do you get, and how much do you think is necessary?
I try to get to bed before midnight and rise early. Six to eight hours a day seems to be ideal, depending on the level of demanding activity. I can function on less, but not well, for extended periods of time. I know the detriments of sleep-deprivation, and it is as unhealthy as anything. Sleep is incredibly important for the healing and building process.

When it comes to relationships, many people just getting into a raw diet have problems because their mates don't want to change. Any comments or suggestions on this?
I would like to believe that love will heal anything. When a couple engages in a shift in interest of diet or lifestyle, it is a hinge for bonding and supporting one another. If only one half of a couple takes a life-changing interest, it can be detrimental to the relationship.

Food is a major issue in most Americans' lives. It is a social and emotional meeting-ground, as well as a very tender spot that can be easily agitated. It is difficult to watch friends and family continue compromised living and health, especially if we have information that we think could liberate them. Hence, there is the common habit of preaching. It's no fun for someone who is not interested.

I know that leading by example is one of the most powerful tools. Avoiding these common pitfalls in a relationship is a delicate dance. Making agreements that serve both people in a relationship is essential. Just as you have the right to change, your partner has the equal right to remain the same.

Ultimately, setting the example of a dietary life change is a telling scenario and may serve as a barometer to determine where both your lives' paths align or diverge.

Do you think it's harder for a man or harder for a woman to eat a raw diet?

I think it's equally easy or challenging for anyone to eat a raw food diet. Constitution, genetic background, and climate, including social climate, seem to have a more potent effect on the success of any exclusive diet. Women and men have different dietary demands that should be attended to accordingly. I am certain that all needs can be met through diverse, plant-based means.

What are your thoughts about the female menstruation cycle on the raw diet?

Discomfort need not be associated with it, and it can be greatly relieved through diet and yoga.

I get my period only several times a year. I have always been very athletic, even before I was hormonally mature, and I was a vegan at a very young age. I believe this partly contributes to this and that I simply have a longer cycle. For the years that I've been into raw foods and yoga, my period has lasted from one to two days. I have had it for as little as a few hours. I rarely even need to use a pad to bleed on. I think tampons are unhealthy, but convenient. My flow is very light.

Do you think it's natural for a woman not to bleed when she is on a raw diet, or should there be blood?

There does not need to be a tremendous amount of blood, but there should be some fluid and tissue. It varies tremendously from woman to woman. All women need to ask themselves if their menstrual cycle feels healthy to know if it is.

Do you have any comments about PMS and the raw diet?

I don't think it's fair or just to make blanket statements in judgment about menstruation and hormone cycles. Each woman has a spectrum of influential factors, with genetic predisposition being a significant dynamic. There is no one answer or correct cycle, though we all represent a rainbow of possibilities.

I've never had cramps or PMS. Pre-Menstrual-Syndrome seems to be a symptom of fluctuating hormones and turmoil. I believe it's widely manufactured, although some women have a really rough go of it at certain points in their cycle.

Thank you for this interview. In closing, is there anything else you would like to add?
Eating a raw food diet for superior health does not make us invincible; it fortifies our resilience. It enables our bodies to recover health more readily. The cooperation of diet, exercise, and spiritual practice accelerates the union of pervasive health and the resonance of true joy. I feel clearer all the time - clear in my body, clear in my mind and clear in my spirit.

Unless an acute health circumstance presses, there is no rush or race to the end. I do not think there is a "finish". We are a constantly evolving process. There are so many details that can improve our health. Beyond our physiological needs are emotional needs and a changing external environment. Be gentle, be sensitive, and be good to yourself.

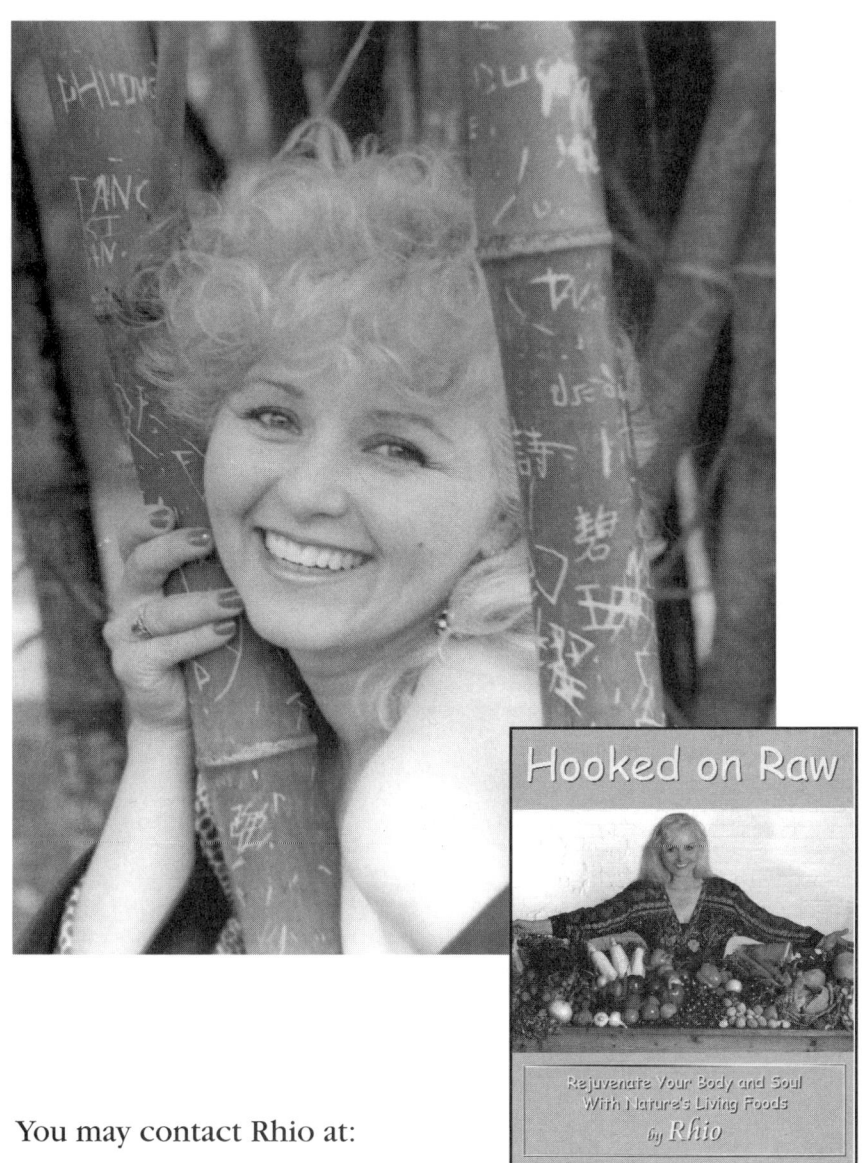

You may contact Rhio at:

Rhio's Raw Energy
Website: www.rawfoodinfo.com
Website: www.fruitandveggielady.com
212-343-1152

Rhio

Rhio is a singer, actress and author, as well as an investigative reporter in the area of health. Rhio, of Hungarian-Cuban descent, raised in the United States, is completely fluent in Spanish. As a performer, she has appeared in over fifty TV shows. Currently, she is completing her third record album for the Latin market. She is also part of an American contemporary singing group that goes by the name of The "Toon" Chicks. The "Toon" Chicks have completed an album which will be out in Fall 2002.

CNN and American Journal have aired stories on the raw food lifestyle featuring Rhio. She is considered an expert in the area of raw and living foods. About five years ago, she started "Rhio's Raw Energy Hotline" on one of her phone lines in New York City where she lives. The hotline, which is updated once each month, provides information for people interested in the raw/live food lifestyle, including upcoming events in the New York area as well as worldwide. The hotline also provides commentary on some of the most pressing health issues of our time: genetic engineering of seeds, food irradiation, electro-magnetic pollution, etc. (212) 343-1152.

Periodically, Rhio hosts a living foods potluck event at her spectacular TriBeCa loft in downtown Manhattan, and from time to time, she offers classes on raw/live gourmet food preparation.

How many years have you been on the raw diet, and what got you into it?
Ten years for sure, and probably fifteen. I started reading the books of Dr. Ann Wigmore when I was a teenager, and they intrigued me. Every time I went on a raw food diet, I always had

lots of energy and felt great. The catalyst that made me stick to it though was the weight I gained (80 pounds) because of a traumatic experience. When I decided to lose the weight, I went on raw juice fasts for a week at a time with lots of exercise. I did this on and off over a six to eight month period. The weight came off, and I started feeling great again. Then I said to myself, "Why don't you just stay on Nature's food for good?" It made good sense to me, so I did.

How was your health when you started the diet?
I've always had good health. Aside from the weight gain, I haven't had any health problems in adulthood except for a few minor ones, like an occasional cold. I also used to get hoarse when I sang a lot. Ever since I started being on raw, even those things don't happen anymore.

When I was carrying around the extra weight though, I did have some problems with the circulation in my hands. That was like a signal to me saying, "Hey, you'd better lose this weight."

Who are some people who have inspired you to do this?
I've read a lot of books, but the ones that really inspired me the most were *The Health Secrets of a Naturopathic Doctor* by M.O. Garten, *Nature's Healing Grasses* by Dr. Kirschner, and Ann Wigmore's books. I was also inspired by Leola Brooks and Lalita Salas at the Ann Wigmore Institute of Puerto Rico. They are the two very loving and dedicated women who inherited the Institute in Puerto Rico when Ann Wigmore died unexpectedly.

Is there any one person who has inspired you the most?
Recently, I've been inspired by the story of Victoria Boutenko, which is recounted in her wonderful book, *The Raw Family*. She and her family of four (mother, father, and two children) came to the United States from Russia approximately twelve years ago. They started living the "good life" and eating the Standard American Diet (SAD). They all eventually became sick, but the final straw for Victoria (the mother) was when

her son was diagnosed with juvenile diabetes. This, she could not accept. The book describes her search for health for her son and the rest of her family. I particularly like the unique way she set about finding the truth. She would be on the lookout for people that appeared to be healthy and vibrant and then she would approach them and ask them what they did to become so healthy. One day, she saw a woman who was glowing with health and asked her the same question. The woman told Victoria that she used to have cancer and had healed herself with a raw food diet. While this information hit Victoria like a ton of bricks, she could nevertheless feel the truth of this simple statement within her soul. The Raw Family is very inspiring to me, and I recently met them. They're wonderful! And of course, they are all healed now.

You've learned so much over the years. What are a few of the most important things you've learned?
I've learned to "walk my talk," which means that I am a dedicated raw food enthusiast. This is my way of life, and I love it and all the benefits that it bestows upon me. I would never tell anyone to follow this path if I were not doing it myself.

In the beginning, of course, I would go back and forth from the raw way to the cooked way and back again to raw. Finally, I discovered that the food itself would help me out. For example, if you say to yourself, "I'm going on high raw (95-100%)," and you manage to do that for an experimental period of three to six months, you will find that when you eat something cooked again, it does not taste as good as you remember. Not only that, but you will also find that now your body is talking to you and it is clearly telling you what kind of energy each type of food gives you. Cooked food always produces a sluggish feeling. But your body will usually not start talking to you (at least not truthfully) until you've done "high raw" for at least three to six months.

While I am enthusiastic about Nature's powerful and healing raw foods, I also realize that there are other factors to consider when trying to maintain or re-gain health. One of the most important of these is mental attitude. A positive (and hopeful) mental attitude goes a long way towards achieving true health. And a sense of gratefulness is also on the top of my list.

Are there any pitfalls that you have learned to watch out for on the raw diet?
Do not make any health teacher into a guru. Think for yourself. Take my teaching and that of others and pass all the information through the fine brain that God has given you, and soon you will discover what will work for you. The raw food diet works for everyone. The problem, however, is in transitioning oneself into it successfully. This transition period may work in one way for one person and in a different way for someone else, because we are all so individual.

So if someone says that he went on raw foods cold turkey, well, that's great, but it might not work for you, so don't let it get you down. For most people, longer transitions in which you first add a lot of raw foods to your present diet and then slowly find satisfying raw substitutes for the cooked foods you presently eat is the better way to go. E A S Y does it.

The fear of losing too much weight is a big pitfall for many people. Any thoughts about that?
Most people who go on a high raw diet find that they lose a lot of weight at first. People who are overweight welcome this. However, some people might lose so much weight that the people around them start to comment about it in a negative way. When this happens, they sometimes become scared; they don't stay the course and they start eating cooked food again. Raw and live foods are not static. These foods get into your system and start to stir and shake things up. What happens is that Nature, in her wisdom, will take you down to the lowest it can in its cleansing process. It's as if Nature is saying to you, "I can't build up anything here until I clear out all of

this garbage first." I believe this is what happens. Then, at some point, while eating the same foods and the same amounts of foods, the body will start to put on weight again. This occurs according to Nature's timetable. I've spoken to many people that this has happened to, including you, Paul.

People with serious health challenges, of course, might benefit from the services of a competent and knowledgeable health care practitioner to guide them through.

Dental problems are another big pitfall. Any thoughts?
I don't believe that most people can thrive on a strict fruitarian diet. I believe that a mixed diet of raw fruits and vegetables, roots, leafy greens, edible weeds, seaweeds, soaked nuts, seeds, and a small to moderate amount of sprouted grains is best. (I prefer the smaller grains like quinoa, amaranth, etc., because the varieties of wheat have been extensively hybridized.)

A fruit diet is very cleansing to the body at first, but it can cleanse too fast. The acidity accumulated in the body's tissues from the person's former diet and lifestyle begins to be released from everywhere in the body, and this acidity also comes out through the tissues in the mouth where it can affect and weaken the teeth. So it's not the fruits themselves that cause damage to the teeth, but the acidity that the fruits are releasing.

For people that are having trouble with their teeth, I would slow down the detox by incorporating more vegetables and sea vegetables into the diet.

Rinse the mouth frequently with a solution of water and Celtic sea salt. Also, to keep tabs on whether there is an acid condition in the mouth, test your saliva with pH paper (but not if you've just recently eaten; it won't be accurate then).
Use an alkaline boost product, if necessary, to try to get your body into a more alkaline state faster. Also, take liquid colloidal minerals, since the amounts of minerals available in our foods may be questionable because so many soils are depleted. Unfortunately, even organic farmers may not be en-

riching their soil to provide more mineral value in the foods. I once worked on an organic farm in Puerto Rico, and their idea of being organic was simply not to spray with pesticides or herbicides. They did very little to enrich the soil. As a consequence, the soil was hard as a rock - not my idea of what organic farming should be. Even so, tests done on organic produce repeatedly find that they have higher nutritional values, including higher mineral content, than conventional produce.

What are your thoughts about mercury fillings, and what would you replace them with?
Mercury fillings should be outlawed. It's unconscionable to put a known toxic substance into people's mouths. Some of the more progressive dentists are substituting with safer materials.

What is your opinion of nuts and seeds?
I love 'em, but I usually soak them first and eat them in moderation. I also sprout the ones that will sprout.

What is your opinion of grains?
Americans eat way too many grain products, much to their detriment. When people first convert to raw, they might also eat too many sprouted grain products to compensate for the unaccustomed feeling of lightness that a fruit and vegetable diet gives them. This may be a necessary step in their transition to raw, but after the initial transition, it is best to eat soaked and sprouted grains only in small to moderate amounts and not everyday.

What is your opinion of a diet of only fruits?
As I stated previously, I have reservations about a strict fruitarian diet. I've noticed that the people who seem to be making a success of fruitarianism are very athletic and get lots of exercise, and they live in sunny climates. I don't know if that has anything to do with it; it is just something that I've observed. Lots of exercise and frequent exposure to sunlight might balance out the sugar of the fruitarian diet.

What is your opinion of sprouts?
Sprouts are wonderful foods. They are easy to grow (even in apartments) and a dependable and economical source of fresh organic food.

What is your opinion of Natural Hygiene?
I agree with many of the principles of Natural Hygiene, but I once subscribed to a Natural Hygiene magazine, and all the recipes it contained involved cooking, so I didn't renew my subscription. I couldn't understand how the editors could recommend a predominantly raw food diet and then publish mostly cooked food recipes.

What is your opinion of supplements?
Low heat processed and food-based supplements are valuable as adjuncts to a raw/live food diet. Some teachers say that we don't need them if we are on a raw/live food diet, but those teachers seem to forget that, in our environment today, we do not have a level playing field. The air is not clean, the water is not clean, and the food is questionable. Many sources of toxicity in the environment are affecting human health. There are high levels of toxins in the atmosphere due to auto exhaust fumes and the by-products of industry.

As I write these few lines, the Mayor and the Department of Health here have just decided to spray extremely toxic pesticides over the population of New York City for the third straight year in a row, supposedly to kill mosquitoes. This abuse has the effect of weakening the immune systems of humans. For these reasons and more, I do believe in getting all the help that we can get.

First, I buy my basic raw/live organic food and then, if I have money left to spend, I will buy genuine food-based, low-heat processed supplements - the best that I can afford.

What is your opinion of eating seasonally?

I absolutely agree with it. The best way is to eat locally grown organic produce. This also benefits the small, local farming communities and saves on the gas needed to transport food over long distances.

Also, locally grown food purchased from farmers' markets is fresher than food shipped across the country, which might be more than a week old before it even gets to your supermarket. A Rutgers University study showed that once produce is picked, it loses 50% of its nutrient value within twenty-four hours.

What is your opinion of fasting?
Fasting is a wonderful tool for cleansing the body of toxicity. I do believe in juice fasting and fasting on the water of big green or yellow water coconuts, such as the ones you find in Puerto Rico or Florida. Unfortunately, these coconuts are not available everywhere in the United States, but maybe, if people start asking for them, the distributors will start bringing them into other areas.

What is your opinion of food combining on a 100% raw diet, and is it necessary?
Except for a few principles that I outline in my book, *Hooked on Raw*, I don't believe that food combining is that essential for a 100% raw food enthusiast. However, if a person has digestive problems or serious health challenges, then I reverse myself and recommend that they follow the food combining guidelines until they are well and their digestion has become strong and resilient. After that, they can either continue to food combine or do some experimenting to see what happens.

What is your opinion of physical exercise?
It is absolutely essential. I suggest that, rather than going to a gym, you find the kind of exercise activity that you personally enjoy doing. That way, you will do it more often, and because it will be enjoyable, you won't have to force yourself to do it. For me it is gardening, dancing, playing tennis, jumping on the

trampoline, and horseback riding. I also love to swim in a clean ocean, but that is getting harder to find.

What is your opinion of wild foods?
If at all possible, add some wild foods to your diet. They are wonderful, very flavorful, and rich in nutrient values.

What are your age, height, and weight? Has your weight changed, or are there any other changes your body has went through?
I don't like the idea of putting a number on people in regards to age, so when pressed, I say that I am an "adult ageless." Many raw food enthusiasts look much younger than their actual years, but the important thing is that they FEEL much younger than their years. People should be vital, productive, and mentally alert until the last day of their lives.

My height is five feet. In the past year, my weight has gone down to 105 pounds, but nobody perceives me as thin because I have a healthy look. Prior to this past year, I weighed 115 pounds.

Did you ever get really sick or have a really bad detox?
No, but I've had some interesting detox experiences. For example, one time when I was fasting on the water of green water coconuts for ten days, around the eighth day I was expelling so much mucous from my chest, I lost my voice. Another thing that happened on this fast was that I started smelling a perfume that I used to wear. At that time, I hadn't worn any perfume for years. But this perfume smell was very strong, and it lasted for about three weeks after the fast was over. So I thought, "Wow, I've detoxed all that perfume." A couple of years later, at the suggestion of a Naturopathic Doctor in California, I went on a three week fast of fresh pomegranate juice (plus some detox herbs that the doctor gave me). Well, guess what? Again the perfume smell came, and it lasted for weeks. And I thought I had gotten rid of it all the first time! But no, there was still more. After that, I've gone on

some other coconut water fasts, and the smell has never returned.

Do you eat 100% raw foods, and if so, for how long? If not, what do you eat that is cooked, and why?
I usually eat 100% raw/live foods, but I'm not perfect. If I'm trying to create a gourmet raw food recipe that is similar to a cooked one, I might take a couple of bites of the cooked one to refresh my memory as to how it tastes. Another exception might be if I get some good foraged wild foods or mushrooms like I did once with Wildman Steve Brill. On one of his walks, we found some Chicken Mushrooms, and he advised me to saute them, because I'm not that knowledgeable about the wild mushrooms and whether you can eat them raw or not. I do eat all the mushrooms that I find in the supermarkets raw, but I never saw a Chicken Mushroom there. Did it taste like chicken? You bet.

What is your average daily diet like? What do you eat, and how often?
I eat all raw and live vegetarian foods of all types. I like a wide variety.

I'm not one of those people who have to have breakfast, lunch, and dinner. I usually eat when I'm hungry. Sometimes I eat three meals a day, but many times two meals a day is enough for me.

What is your favorite food?
As funny as it might seem to some newcomers to raw, I have become very fond of the "heavy" greens. By heavy greens, I mean the collards, kale, Swiss chard, beet tops, and wild greens. I put a tasty marinade on them, toss, and eat.

I don't marinate greens overnight myself, but I suggest doing that in my book because it will help newcomers adapt to the flavor in the beginning. I also add other things to the basic greens recipe that can vary the flavor and make them more tasty and palatable. It is my goal to develop at least one hundred different marinated greens recipes, so that people will never get tired of or bored with their greens.

Out of all of the foods, what do you think is the most important?

Because of the lower availability of oxygen in our cities (8-10% instead of 21%), I would say that leafy greens are the most important, including leaf lettuces, collards, kale, Swiss chard, spinach, and wild leafy greens.

How are your health and energy?

The best they've ever been.

How much sleep do you get, and how much do you think is necessary?

On a daily basis, I only seem to need five to six hours. However, I have noticed that from time to time I sleep more, especially when I'm on vacations or away from my regular home life. The number of hours that a person needs is an individual matter. From studies that have been done, it seems that the average for most people is eight hours per night.

Have you noticed any mental changes on the raw diet?

There is more mental clarity, and I have many moments of intuition, which, when acted upon, turn out to be correct.

When it comes to relationships, many people just getting into a raw diet have problems because their mates don't want to change. Any comments or suggestions on this?

It depends on the person. Some people could probably live with a person who doesn't want to go the raw way. My partner didn't want to do it, and that was the primary reason I created my gourmet raw recipes - I was trying to entice him into it. It did work partially, and for a very long time he was 70% raw. And that helped to make it work between us. But recently he decided to go 100% raw on his own. A man in Atlanta, Georgia, the husband of a couple that went raw, had inspired him. I find that amusing, because all this time I've been writing, lecturing, preparing raw food, and doing all that I do, and it didn't motivate him, but it took only a few words from someone else to make him want to go all the way to 100%. But I'm really grateful for those few words.

Do you think it is harder to eat a raw diet today, or was it harder to do years ago?
I don't think the time frame really matters. It's a matter of being addicted to cooked food flavors and figuring out how to get over it. On second thought, it may be more difficult now because we are addicted not only to cooked food, but also to factory food or "food artifacts."

Do you think it is harder for a man than it is for a woman to eat a raw diet?
I think it is probably easier for a woman, because women just generally seem to have more health awareness. For example, when I go to health spas and even to the raw food institutes, who do I see there? Predominantly women. Why? One reason is women's vanity. We just want to look good, feel good, and look younger. And somehow, we intuit that the way to get these things is through diet and lifestyle.

What is your opinion about the female menstruation cycle on the raw diet?
For me, it went down to less than half a day per month. Do you think it is natural for a woman not to bleed when she is on a raw diet, or should there be blood? There should be a small flow, perhaps two to three pads. I don't believe in using tampons. There has to be a little bit of blood there in case of pregnancy (the germ plasm has a need for nourishment), but certainly not the huge flows (six to seven days) that is considered normal in our society.

Any comments about PMS and the raw diet?
You don't get PMS on the raw diet.

Any comments about pregnancy and the raw diet?

The raw diet makes everything easier for the mother. But don't begin a raw food diet during pregnancy, because if you do, your body will be going through a cleanse at an inappropriate time. However, adding lots more raw food during this time is good.

Where do you see the raw food movement heading in the future?
I believe it's going to go more mainstream, as unbelievable as that may seem right now. It will be a process for people where they might become vegetarian first and then make a transition to raw. The oncoming scandal concerning meat will spur it on, as it did in England a few years ago. When the Mad Cow Disease spread in England, a few million people instantly became vegetarians. I think something like that is heading here in the near future. They can't hide nvCJD (the human equivalent of Mad Cow Disease) under the cover of Alzheimer's forever. The truth will out.

Thank you for this interview. In closing, is there anything else you would you like to add?
Well, I want to thank you too for inviting me to do this interview. Your first book was wonderful, and I know that this new book will be a success, too. I particularly enjoyed the part where you said that you found your way to health by noticing what the doctors would tell you to do and then doing the opposite. That was hilarious. You did it the hard way by trial and error.

I invite people to visit my website where I have placed a great deal of information about the raw lifestyle. It is www.rawfoodinfo.com. I have compiled Directories which make it easier for raw food people in many states and countries to find each other. Also, there is an Events Calendar by state and country and a "Real Letters from Real People" section that is very interesting, precisely because real people wrote the letters.

Come visit sometime, and God bless you!

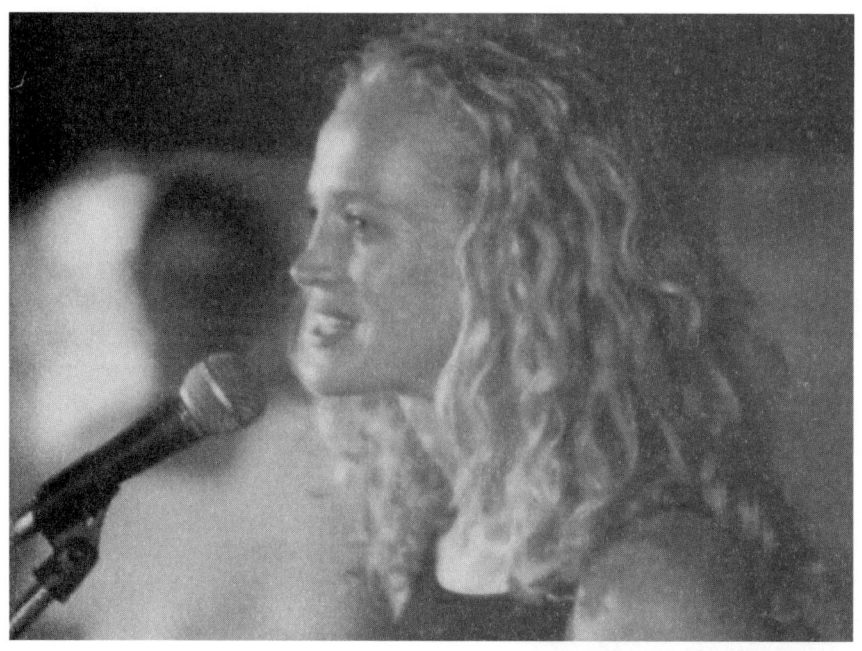

You may contact Annie at:

Annie Jubb
Jubb's Longevity, Inc.
508 East 12th Street
New York, NY 10009
E-mail: excellenceinc@earthlink.net
or annie@lifefood.com
212-358-8068

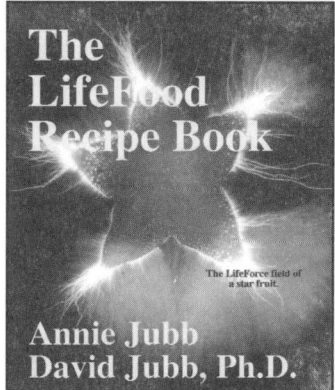

Annie Jubb

Annie Jubb is the co-author of *The LifeFood Recipe Book, Colloidal Biology* and *Secrets of an Alkaline Body*, along with five other books on Whole Brain Functioning, her training program co-created with David Jubb, Ph.D., her partner of fifteen years. Whole Brain Functioning (WBF) training is adventure-based experiential learning that creates deep resource states of consciousness through fire walking, sweat lodges, and adventure ropes courses. Annie is known to her clients as a shaman, a healer, a spiritual leader, an amazing speaker, and an expert on the body-mind-spirit connection.

LifeFood Nutrition is a major component of WBF. It is the use of food as medicine and the inner-standing that there is only one real dis-ease, toxicity and enervation, which is the lack of electrics in the body. Annie has guided thousands of people through Jubb's 14-Day LifeFood Nutritional Fast. This program is enormously successful because it is easy to follow. The healthy person will look years younger after the Fast, and the health-challenged individual can begin the necessary regeneration process when provided with the vital electrics and nutrition needed. LifeFood Nutrition consists of fresh raw organic fruits and vegetables with soaked or ground nuts and seeds, along with some fermented foods and cold-pressed oils.

How many years have you been on the raw diet, and what got you into it?
I call it a Lifefood diet. I've been on a Lifefood diet for more than twelve years. It has been more than twelve years since I've eaten anything that would struggle to get away: meat, fish, fowl, or the eggs of their unborn offspring. It has been a

transformation of spirit to continue.

Why did you start eating a healthier diet?
I got into this way of eating by discovering enzymes and thus perfected the ultimate healing diet. The news of enzymes was compelling and irrevocable. Once I learned about enzymes, it was all over for cooked, denatured, processed food in my diet. I felt a strong connection to starches and had a long withdrawal from starches before I felt free from them. I decided to become a vegetarian first and let go of cooked food within a few months.

What is so special about the Lifefood diet?
The Lifefood diet focuses on cleansing the body. This diet is the top of the mountain for beginning the cleansing process. It is a low-glycemic diet that is ideal for everyone. Eating a Lifefood diet is the way to heal from all diseases. The 14-day Lifefood nutritional fast is the ultimate healing diet to clear debris from the deep places in the body, especially the liver, and gallbladder.

Who are some people who have inspired you to do this?
Dr. Ann Wigmore was an original spirit. She inspired me. I read one of her recipe books and never went back.

Is there any one person who has inspired you the most?
Dr. David Jubb, my longtime partner. He keeps me updated on the latest understandings in health from the true renegades in science and medicine. He's years ahead of his time.

You have learned so much over the years. What are a few of the most important things you have learned?
Starches are the scourge of humanity and the root issue of many diseases.

Most people are riddled with gallstones and have a congested liver. My program is the surgery-free option to clear this matter easily from the body.

Most symptoms of the body can be relieved within days of my 14-day Lifefood nutritional fast program. Blood sugar normalizes within twenty-four hours!

The most important things in life are stated well in the Hawaiian culture: You only really need three things: something to do, something to look forward to, and someone to share it with.

How can people avoid the pitfalls that they might encounter on the raw diet?
The key is to surround yourself with likeminded individuals. The people you share time with will either empower you to unimaginable heights or spiral you down to nothing. Many people will go their whole lives without ever realizing the direct cause and effect of this, since it is so close to them. Practice Satsang: keeping company with likeminded individuals.

Weight loss is a big pitfall for many people. Any thoughts about that?
People will often go all the way down with their weight before they become able to gain back a good weight. Why? Much of the density that people sport is particalized starches striated within the musculature of the body tissue. In other words, there's bread and pasta (mucus) packed around the cells and right throughout the body, along with rancid fats, indigestible proteins, enzyme-resistant protein chains from animal flesh and pasteurized milk, mucus, insipid pus, and lots of other garbage from meals such as chips, canned food, boxed crackers, cereals, and pasta. This creates a false sense of bigness. This is a pre-diabetic condition. A diet high in starches and animal protein will plump up a person, while slowly packing the organs with stored material that often ends up being the death of a person.

Large muscles can be truly gained only through weight-bearing strength training, such as weightlifting or any physical exercise that is anaerobic. Of course, true good health is obtained through a combination of the above along with aerobic activity.

Dental problems are another big pitfall. Do you have any thoughts about that?
I had all my metal amalgam fillings removed several years ago, and I wish I'd done it better and sooner. I recommend removing them in most cases, except when a person is in very poor health. Always ask the dentist for a dental dam. I also recommend that people take 5,000 to 10,000 mg of Vitamin C during the days prior to the amalgam removal and throughout, or use a good antioxidant like Pycnogenol.

Good dental hygiene is very important. Brushing twice a day, flossing, using a tongue cleaner and herbal mouthwash are all vital to good dental health.

What is your opinion of nuts and seeds?
I love them. Nuts and seeds are essential for the cold pressed oils they provide to lubricate the body and make the blood more slippery.

More use can be made of fatty nuts like brazil, walnut and pine nuts. It's great to blend them up into a milk. That is my favorite food everyday! Seeds such as sesame, pumpkin, hemp and flax provide essential fatty acids like no others! We need these fats for good brain functioning. The protein provided in nuts and seeds are superior to animal proteins in that they are living, as evidenced in sprouting. They are easiest to assimilate when soaked or ground to a fine meal for easy digestion.

What is your opinion of grains?
Most grain should be avoided for ideal health. For the unwell person, they should be avoided totally. All grains are starchy and high-glycemic. These foods complicate the job of the already taxed liver and pancreas.

Forcing the production of insulin to slow down speedy

blood sugar is the cause of most modern illness. All noodles, crackers, pasta, wheat, corn, rice, potatoes (and products made from them), and all packaged cereals are in this starch category.

What is your opinion of an all fruit diet?
This is a wonderful practice and should be practiced often. By resorting to seasonal local fruits, one acclimatizes and bioregionalizes very quickly. Pollen allergies often subside when one fasts upon fresh fruits of the season. Is this a good diet for one's lifetime? Not for longer than a few months, and it depends upon one's health. A person who is very sick and obese can go for many months purifying upon seasonal fruits (fruit: coming from a flower). People who live in cities must have dark leafy greens with their fruit to combat the pollution in the air they breathe, so I recommend lots of dark green juices for those people. If you live in a luscious environment, perhaps in the jungle and near a waterfall, then by all means fast upon fruit for many moons.

What is your opinion of sprouts?
I love the good young energy of sprouts! Grain sprouts make otherwise starchy high-glycemic messes into fruit-like sugars! Grass sprouts are full of oxygen and chlorophyll. They are simply the perkiest little tasty guys around.

What is your opinion of supplements?
Whole food vitamin/mineral supplements have a measurable life force and thus qualify for Lifefood nutrition. We love the potentiated nutrition found in herbal and whole food supplements and have forwarded them to our clients for years. We carry only these high quality supplements at our clinic store, Jubb's Longevity, Inc.

Pharmaceutical grade vitamins are usually inorganic and are often stored in organ tissue. They should be avoided.

What is your opinion of eating seasonally?

You should eat seasonally and locally as much as possible. I've already mentioned how this helps heal seasonal allergies and to acclimatize oneself.

What is your opinion of fasting?
I'm the queen of fasting. I love it more than eating. I've promoted my 14-day Lifefood nutritional fast for more than a decade and taught tens of thousands of people how to clear gallstones and toxins from their bodies non-surgically and without drugs. Fasting heals the root of the problem. I have yet to meet a person who doesn't have gallstones.

What is your opinion of food combining on a 100% raw diet, and is it necessary?
Of course it is. Try eating banana with soaked oat groats and look out! Have a little Kim Chee then, and you'll be sorry.
It's important to eat sensibly. I've experienced a personal case of gluttony on Lifefood many times (I'm sorry to say). Eating too much food or eating a gaseous combination is always a regrettable move.

What is your opinion of physical exercise?
Gotta have it. If I exercise less than about two hours a day, then I'm one cranky dakini! I love to be in the outdoors. Even in the wilds of NYC, I ride my bike, roller blade, run, walk miles and miles, and get to the gym and do a good Astanga yoga class.

What is your opinion of wild foods?
These are the highest vibe foods around. Wild-grown food has become stronger and more resilient because it has had to fight off natural enemies: mold, fungus, yeast, parasites, bacteria, rodents, etc. Its life-force is measurably greater (see Kirlean photography in my book), and it possesses many more minerals and vitamins as a result of its robust good health.

What are your age, height, and weight? Has your weight changed, or were there any other changes your body went through? How did you handle it?
I don't do age, though thanks for asking. I am five feet nine inches and weigh 117 pounds almost always except when fasting, when I get down to 110 pounds.
I've always been thin, although when I found out about enzymes and jumped onto Lifefood, I weighed about five pounds more and wore a C-cup bra. I actually started running about two years before that time and had dropped most of my body fat by that point, though losing the last part of my weight did shrink my breasts. They look nice and they are firm, as always happens when you lose weight through Lifefood. You just look better and not fat.

Did you ever get really sick or have a really bad detox?
I didn't, although I designed my fasts around those that reported feeling sick at times. Now most people report feeling great throughout my Lifefood nutritional fast.

Do you eat 100% raw foods, and if so, for how long? If not, what do you eat that is cooked, and why?
My everyday diet is all Lifefood. On special occasions and just for fun, sometimes I eat lightly steamed vegetables with my mostly Lifefood meal.

What is your average daily diet like? What do you eat, and how often?
I consume Lifefood blended or juiced beverages during the day. Sometime around 8:00 p.m., I feel like having dinner and usually have two or three different salads with vegetables. I love avocado, olives, tomato, cucumber, asparagus, and zucchini with raw oils such as olive and hemp or a great dressing, and I eat a little raw goat cheese. I eat dehydrated food like flax seed crackers and breads made from flax seeds as well as luscious preparations that I sell at my store, LONGEVITY. I eat

tons of seasonal fruits, often in juice, smoothie, or soup form.

What is your favorite food?
Right now, it's cherries. I eat a bag of Cascadian Farms frozen black sweet cherries every day, and have for about three years.

Of all foods, what do you think is the most important?
Dark leafy greens! It's the most important food for Americans and all modern world people. Most everyone who comes to my clinic is magnesium-deficient. Magnesium is found abundantly in all dark leafy green vegetables, algae, and fruit. Magnesium is nature's tranquilizer. It allows over 300 different detoxification pathways of the body to open and clear toxins that have been on hold for many years. This is the medicine of the future! I am a huge magnesium fan and encourage everyone to increase his or her magnesium intake. In 1900, most Americans took in about 500 mg. daily. Now people take in only 125 mg. daily - a huge deficit.

Eat your greens, juice them, blend them into great soups. It will save your life.

How are your health and energy?
Wonderful. I almost always work too hard, and I gain a spurt in health whenever I slow down. All in all, if my mood is good, so is my health. Emotion is always the thing that I have to be careful of. I think too much and feel so deeply that it is sometimes to my disadvantage. Strong spiritual practice is my good medicine for this, and lots of green drinks!

How much sleep do you get, and how much do you think is necessary?
Usually, I run on sleep according to my sleeping place. In NYC, I sleep between seven and twelve hours a day most of the time, depending on how much spiritual work I am doing. I sleep less as I go west: in Los Angeles and Seattle, I usually need seven or eight hours a day. In Hawaii, I sleep six or

seven hours. This changes dramatically when I am working. During a training of seven to fourteen days, I'll typically sleep three to five hours and wake up with a list of things to do: a complete agenda of what to teach, an idea of what specific teaching a participant needs, and so on.

If I have a four month run of trainings, lectures, and workshops with lots of travel, I'll sleep little and lightly, getting a good twelve hour sleep once a week. I love to dream, and I can't go without my nighttime travels for long.

Have you noticed any mental changes on the raw diet?
I'm sharper and more alert, both in my day and in the dreamtime. Lifefood naturally turns to face nature, so nature arises within you. It is your natural state to be empathic, psychic, telepathic. These natural traits arise spontaneously within you as you incorporate 80% Lifefood in your diet. It's really stunning how easy it is to get a huge jolt toward enlightenment simply by eating Lifefood. The simple teachings are often the most trying.

Many people just beginning a raw diet have problems because their mates do not want to change. Do you have any comments or suggestions? What are your thoughts about relationships?
Quite frankly, it is nearly impossible for me to be in a relationship with someone who is on a cooked/meat diet. I've tried to be in one because of a huge spiritual connection and thought it could work, and it was too much for me. A relationship is such a blend of the two of you that there simply must be common ground. For me, meat-eating and cooked food (more than, say, between 10-20%) are too harsh. That's how I feel now, and how I've felt for some time.

Life is a balance. Sharing an existence is so special and precious and rare to find, it's time you must be picky and encourage the environment that is ideal for you. Whatever heaven on earth is for you, you must create it.

Has your opinion towards sex changed over the years?
No. I love sex and always have. Since the time I became sexually active until today, I have reveled in long and passionate lovemaking sessions with my mate. I enjoy a monogamous relationship, serial monogamy, I guess you call it, with my partner and am always building upon our prior sessions. Loving, daily monogamous lovemaking is the best combination of meditation, exercise, and couplehood.

What are your thoughts about the female menstruation cycle?
On a Lifefood diet, your moon will normalize, and the flow will decrease to its normal nomadic flow. In other words, you will bleed only a little bit (a tablespoon or so per month). For a sexually active woman, I've found that this is very good, and it assures the woman that her body is working with her in her effort to control pregnancy.

Do you think it's natural for a woman to bleed when she is on a raw diet?
It's not uncommon for a woman on Lifefood to bleed very lightly during her moon. However, if a woman who did not have great health and had uterus issues before she changed to a Lifefood diet is not bleeding, she should seek health counsel. Sometimes the uterus lining is stagnant and should be brought down with herbs. Exercise is always good for a healthy immune system.

Any comments about PMS and the raw diet?
Lifefood - a refinement of the raw food diet - is the best diet for PMS. Without fail, I get comments from many women on Lifefood who love the freedom from PMS that they have now.

Any comments about pregnancy and the raw diet?
Enjoy a healthy diet rich in the bounty of nature. Eat from this

richness and eat it in this living whole lifeforce-rich goodness. Pregnancy on Lifefood (eating a full range of foods) is seeking nature as your midwife. Giving birth in the cull (with the embryonic sack intact) is the gift from nature. Birth is easy, and as in the case of all animals, works hydraulically.

Thank you for this interview. In closing, is there anything else you would you like to add?
Lifefood nutrition is fresh raw fruits, vegetables, seeds, and nuts grown organically and in season, along with some fermented food that is properly combined for easy digestion. Green is clean! Eat and drink your greens.

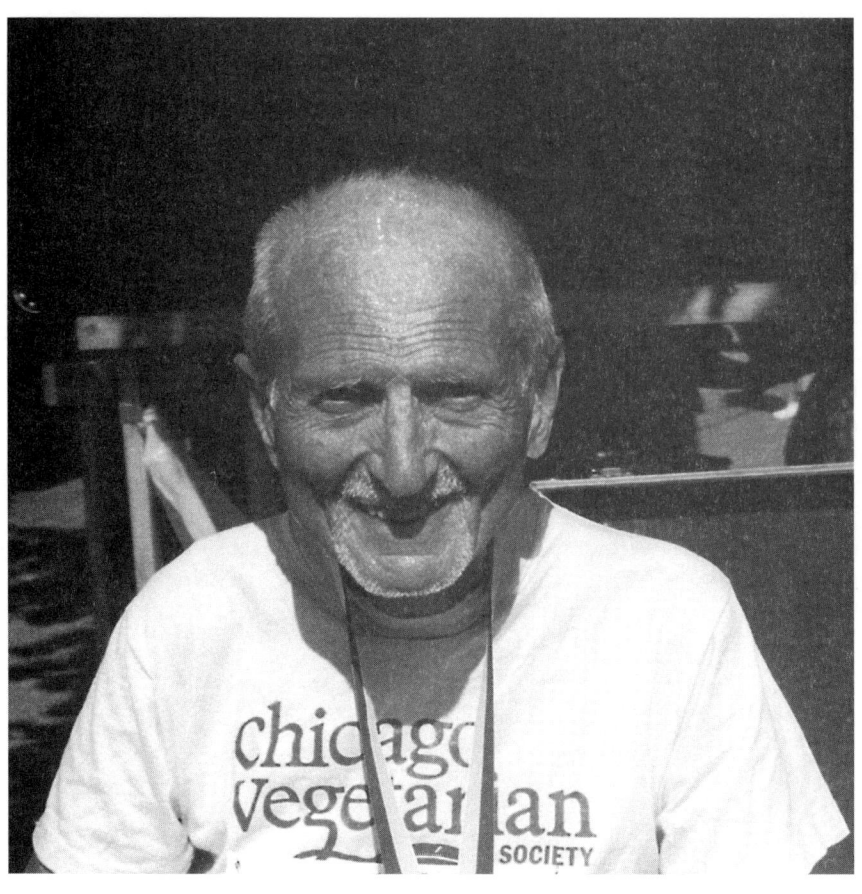

You may contact Arne at:
** See note at the end of the interview.

Arne Wingqvist

My name is Arne Wingqvist. I am a Swedish male born in 1919 and still going strong. I started with a vegetarian bill of fare in 1931. After about ten years, I skipped the milk products. Since about 1985, I've been eating mostly fresh fruit, nuts, seeds, and fresh uncooked vegetables, mostly green leafy ones, veganic-organic, if possible.

My wife and I have five children between the ages of thirty and forty as well as five grandchildren between the ages of nine months and six years. All ten are vegetarians/vegans.

In the mid-1940s, I became a life-time member of the Swedish Vegetarian Society and The Nordic Society against Painful Experiments on Animals.

After World War II, in July 1945, I joined the Swedish Red Cross. I was in a convoy of about ten to twelve trucks that transported medicines and provisions to Prague, the capital of Czechoslovakia in those days. After some time, I changed over to World Y.M.C.A. (Young Men's Christian Association). We worked with displaced persons, i.e., people from former East European countries who had fled to West Germany and lived in refugee camps waiting to be cleared to go to their relatives all over the world.

When this task was finished, I was employed as a civilian in the U.S. Army in West Germany as a German/English translator. I returned to Sweden in 1947 and stayed there until 1951, working with the Thomas Cook & Son Travel Agency in Stockholm.

In 1951, I moved to New York City for some months, then to Minneapolis, Minnesota, and later to San Antonio, Texas. There, I studied Natural Hygiene with the late Dr. Herbert M. Shelton, who was the most outstanding representative of our days of Natural Hygiene and fasting.

In 1952, I went to Los Angeles and Hollywood, California and stayed there until 1954. While living in California, I visited Sweden to participate in the IVU Congress 1953, which was held in Sigtuna, the oldest town in Sweden. I was invited to speak about vegetarianism in the U.S.A. After the congress, I returned to California for another year.

In the summer of 1954, I moved back to Sweden. That year, I took part in the "Great Fasting Walkathon" from Gothenburg to Stockholm. We fasted for seventeen days, from August 1 to August 17. Our group consisted of eleven men, and we only drank water. The first ten days we walked 50 kilometers (about 31 miles) per day. During the last seven days, medical doctors examined us, taking all kinds of tests. They told us we were in better shape than we were before we started. The average weight loss was about nine to ten kilograms. We were on the front pages of many newspapers in Sweden for fourteen days. We had television in those days. The press in many countries all over the world also wrote about the Fasting Walkathon.

In 1954, I also started The National Association Against Tobacco in Sweden and was elected charter president. In those days, about 50% of adults were smokers; today, in 1998, less than 25% are smokers.

In 1955, I went to North Queensland, Australia. I was part owner of a banana plantation on the Athertone Tableland, 100 kilometers north of Cairns. I stayed there about a year before returning to Sweden, where I married and was busy raising our five kids until 1986.

After all these years in Sweden, I moved to Belgium in 1986 and stayed there until August 1988, when I moved to the French Riviera. I live just outside Nice, usually spending the summer months in Sweden with my family and the winter months in Thailand, or in other places around or south of the equator, where "the sun spends the winter."

During my travels, I give lectures about vegetarianism/veganism. In 1997, I organized an international bicycle tour in Sweden all the way from Kiruna in the North, above the Artic Circle, to Stockholm, the capital of Sweden, for a length of 1,410 kilometers (about 881 miles). There were seven of us altogether. Some participated part of the way, according to the agreement at the time of registration, but two other participants and I and made it all the way to the finish. Among them was Sigrid De Leo, EVU Secretary. During the trip, we only had water to drink and only fresh fruit, nuts, and fresh, raw, vegetables to eat. We wanted to prove that on this bill of fare, one could achieve a strenuous workout over a long period, from July 15 to August 2 (19 days), and still feel in top shape. During the trip, we gave lectures to people in the towns and villages we passed through. Newspapers interviewed us, and I was interviewed on the radio as well.

I have been a strict vegetarian/vegan since 1931, always eating a minimum of 50% fresh, uncooked, vegetables at meals. Eventually, I stopped destroying the food by cooking and started eating everything fresh and unadulterated instead.

My sixty-seven years of experience of healthy living and healthy eating have taught me that uncooked food is the best for me. Fruit and vegetables, veganic-organic if possible, come ready from Nature, contain all we need, take a minimum of time to prepare, and require a minimum of time for washing up after the meal. It will suit most people, as it suits me. If you wish to try it out, I advise you to do it very carefully. At the very least, it helps you to keep the waistline from bulging out as the years pass by.

I have been invited to give a lecture at the IVU Congress which runs January 4-10, 1999 in Chiang Mai. The title of the lecture is "Dining Well the Veggie Way." I am looking forward to meeting you all. Before arriving in Chiang Mai, I will stop in Kuala Lumpur, Malaysia, for about ten days to visit friends and give some lectures at the Vegetarian Society. After the Congress, I might go to Singapore and Australia.

Please overlook the length of my introduction, but I have lived a long, happy, vegetarian/vegan life, of which this is only a very compressed summary.

Essene Gospel of Peace - a Third Century manuscript:
"Kill neither men, nor beasts, not yet the food which goes into your mouth. For if you eat living food, the same will quicken you, but if you kill your food, the dead food will kill you also... For everything which kills your foods, kills your bodies also... And your bodies become what your foods are..."

Yours in Friendship,
Arne Wingqvist

How many years have you been on the raw diet, and what got you into it?
I started with lacto-vegetarian food in 1931. At least 60-70% of my diet was fresh, raw food. Soon afterward, I cut down on the little lacto that I used, and some years later, I left it entirely.

The most important reason for going raw to me was my respect for animals and nature. The health aspect, one can forget about, because if you live right, perfect health comes to you as a bonus. That is Nature's way to "thank you" for obeying her laws. Animals can't talk; that is why we must talk for the animals.

How was your health when you started the diet?
Perfect.

Who are some people who have inspired you to do this?
There was a man named Edvin Ahlqvist. He was well known as a boxing promoter for Ingemar Johansson, who won the Swedish world heavyweight boxing championship by beating

Floyd Patterson in New York City on June 25, 1959, by a knockout in the third round. Ingemar Johansson later moved to Florida, where he has a motel. Edvin Ahlqvist was a sports journalist by profession and was employed by Bernarr MacFadden in New York City. In the early 1930's, he had returned to Sweden. He had picked up the ideas of vegetarianism, and when I met him in 1931, he spoke about how good it was to give up meat, fish, fowl, and eggs. It was easy for me because I did not like meat and fish. I also read books and found out by myself.

Is there any one person who has inspired you the most?
You ask for one person, but I have many. I will name people who have been very important in the "natural health movement": The Danish Doctor Kirstine Nolfi in Humlebeck, Denmark, Are Waerland in Sweden, Dr. Herbert M. Shelton of San Antonio, Texas. I studied "The Natural Hygenic System" with him in 1951-52. I have met Dr. Bernard Jensen at his retreat in the San Bernardino area near Los Angeles, California. I met Ann Wigmore in Boston, Massachusetts and in Stockholm in the 1970s. I have read most of her books.
I have also known English, German, Swiss, Swedish, Finnish, and Norwegian well known personages. They were forerunners and pioneers in making vegetarian ideas what they are today.

You have learned so much over the years. What are a few of the most important things you have learned?
That I still have very much to learn. Not to push other people into it. That everything except fresh raw food is junk food and poisons you. There is nothing better than 100% raw food. When I see people in the supermarkets with their shopping carts, I see a straight line to the hospital.

Are there any pitfalls that you have learned to watch out for on the raw diet?
No, except to watch out for people who do not know what they're talking about when they argue that you cannot live on

raw food and cannot live without meat. That is of course a lot of "B.S."

Weight loss is a big pitfall for many people. Any thoughts about that?
On raw food, you keep the weight which is the correct weight for you. In the U.S.A., over 50% of the population or even more are overweight. They would all reach their correct weight on raw food, and those who are underweight would gain weight.

Dental problems are another big pitfall. Any thoughts?
Dental problems will stop. Of course, you have to see the dentist to get cavities filled, etc., but when that is done, there should be no problems.

What are your thoughts about mercury fillings, and what would you replace them with?
They ought to be replaced, preferably with gold fillings. I had all mine changed in 1945 to gold fillings.

What is your opinion of nuts and seeds?
They should be eaten sparingly. The liver, for example, can take about four to five almonds daily. All dried fruit, nuts, and seeds should be soaked between six and twenty-four hours. Sprouted seeds, etc., are best.

What is your opinion of grains?
They are no food for man. Stay away.

What is your opinion of sprouts?
Sprouts are excellent!

What is your opinion of Natural Hygiene?
I studied Natural Hygiene with Doctor Herbert M. Shelton in San Antonio, Texas back in 1951-1952. He was a marvelous man, the greatest man of the 20th century. But in those days, raw food was not in vogue like it is today.

What is your opinion of supplements?
Supplements are not necessary and should not be used too much. Getting what you need through raw food is best. You must watch your Vitamin B12 reading. In an all raw food intake, we even usually get enough of the polyunsaturated fatty acids (PUFAs), of which two are essential – Linoleic acid and Alpha-linolenic acid.

What is your opinion of eating seasonally?
I usually buy fruits and vegetables which are "in season." I try to buy produce that is grown locally.

What is your opinion of fasting?
Fasting is very good for those who need it – i.e., almost everybody. Just drink water to keep the thirst away. No enemas. No exercise. It is important to break the fast very carefully. Do not return to your old diet after the fast, but change over to a more strict diet.

What is your opinion of food combining on a 100% raw diet, and is it necessary?
If you eat a mono fruit meal, the stomach knows how to digest it. If you eat a fruit cocktail, blame yourself for the problems it causes. For salad plates, make it simple, not mixed too much, and never with fruit except for veggie fruits - i.e., tomatoes, cucumbers, etc. Avocado also goes well with a salad plate.

What is your opinion of physical exercise?
It is a must! Walking, jogging, skiing, swimming, etc. are very good. A fast walk or jog for twenty to thirty minutes a day keeps your heart and lungs, as well as your whole body, young.

What is your opinion of wild foods?
Can you get those today? Berries and whatever you can get are very good. You can pick herbs, etc., but wild veggie food is hard to find.

What are your age, height, and weight? Has your weight changed, or are there any other changes your body has gone through? How did you handle it?
I was born 1919. Before September 8, 1997, my height was 181 centimeters; after that date, it became 171 centimeters. I had a terrible bicycle accident that almost crushed some vertebrae, etc., and I lost 10 centimeters in height. I could hardly walk more than 300-400 meters for two and a half to three years. Now I take long walks and walk rather fast. I ride a bicycle and have a very special gymnastic program, the best in the world.

I have never had any problems with my weight. But other people have problems with my weight. They say I am grossly underweight. But remember that BMI, etc. is calculated based on meat-eaters, not on healthy people. I may say that I am, in certain respects, stronger than the average man over forty and many men who are even younger.

Did you ever get really sick or have a really bad detox?
Yes. But not so bad that I couldn't live through it. I did not have much of a detox, though, because I had been fasting very often in earlier days, twice for four weeks, and numerous times any number of days after that. In 1954, I took part in a 530 kilometer fasting walkathon, only drinking water. Eleven of us walked about 50 kilometers per day for ten days, and on top of that we fasted for another seven days. In 1997, I bicycled 881 miles in nineteen days, sightseeing en route. There were seven of us, and three of us made it all the way, eating only fresh fruit, fresh raw vegetables, and nuts and seeds. I was seventy-eight years old at the time, and the other two, a woman from Switzerland and a man from Stockholm, were fifty-three years old.

Do you eat 100% raw foods, and if so, for how long?
Yes, 100% raw for about eighteen to twenty years. But re-

member that I have been eating 60-70% raw food since 1931.

What is your average daily diet like? What do you eat, and how often?
My breakfast is a mono fruit meal. My lunch is a mono fruit meal, two or three bananas, or one or two apples, or a mango, or some oranges or grapefruits, etc. I try to stick to fruit in season. My dinner is a salad plate with plenty of lettuce and other leafy colorful veggies, with an avocado, tomato, cucumber, etc.

What is your favorite food?
Fresh fruit.

Of all foods, what do you think is the most important?
Veganic-organanic fruit and veggies.

How are your health and energy?
Excellent!

How much sleep do you get, and how much do you think is necessary?
Five to six hours. How much you need depends on many things, such as age, surroundings, work, etc.

Have you noticed any mental changes?
Not many, except my mentality is getting stronger.

When it comes to relationships, many people just getting into a raw diet have problems because their mates don't want to change. Any comments or suggestions on this?
I have never had any trouble. My peace of mind forbids me to waste my mental powers on quarrels. My wife likes her cooked food - vegetarian/vegan, of course - and I do not give two hoots about it.

Has your attitude towards sex changed over the years?
No. The more, the better.

Do you think it is harder for a woman to eat a raw diet than it is for a man?
No.

What are your thoughts about the female menstruation cycle?
The raw diet is good for women. Troubles usually disappear.

Do you think it's natural for a woman not to bleed when she is on a raw diet, or should there be blood? Either way you answer, please explain why.
There should be no blood. No cooked food, salt, etc. - no blood, or just very little.

Any comments about PMS and the raw diet?
In many cases, the raw diet will make PMS disappear.

Any comments about pregnancy and the raw diet?
The raw diet is good for both mother and child. There is no shortage of milk when the baby is born.

Thank you for this interview. In closing, is there anything else you would you like to add?
Yes. I would like to present a discussion of the effect of raw food on the world community, the environment, the world economy, etc.

Talk given by Arne Wingqvist (Sweden) in Thailand on January 6, 1999. Recorded and reproduced by David Román.

Introduction: I'm honored to be introducing the speaker for this session to all of you. The speaker this morning has been a vegetarian for many, many years and has been a fruitarian for the past twelve to fifteen years. During his period of being a fruitarian, he hasn't eaten any cooked food; he just eats fruits. Four years ago, he came here for a walkathon in Thailand. He is about 80 years old now, and he is active and as strong as ever. So this morning, he will speak to you about being a healthy fruitarian. I'd like to introduce you to Arne Wingqvist.

Arne Wingqvist: Thank you, friends. I welcome you all to this little lecture on fasting. The title is, *Fasting According to the Principles of the Natural Hygiene System* taught by the late Dr. Herbert M. Shelton of San Antonio, Texas, U.S.A. I will give you a little introduction to Dr. Shelton, from the book, *FIT FOR LIFE*. Many of you have read it. There it says: "One of the most world respected and notable Natural Hygienists of our time is Dr. Herbert M. Shelton, now retired, who from 1928 until 1981 led a 'health school,' including a clinic, laboratories, and teaching programs, in San Antonio, Texas. Dr. Shelton is generally considered to be the greatest authority on Natural Hygiene philosophy, principles, and practice. He produced a wealth of literature with new findings, and added more to the science and art of Natural Hygiene than any other person. In Dr. Shelton's own words, 'The laws of nature, the truths of the universe, the principles of science, are just as certain, as fixed and immutable in relation to health as they are in relation to all things else. Natural Hygiene is a branch of biology which investigates and applies the conditions upon which life and health depend, and the means by which health is sustained in all its virtue and purity, and restored when it has been lost or impaired.'"

I had the pleasure - I would say the fortune - to be a student of Dr. Shelton's Health School in 1951-1952. I consider that period to be one of the most valuable in all my life.

Fasting: In English you have "breakfast," that is, you "break the fast." You eat your last meal at night and then you sleep all night and in the morning you take breakfast: you break the fast you've had during the night. It's the same wording in French (jeûne et déjeuner) and in Spanish, etc. Fasting means to abstain from food, except water. Water is also food, but you abstain from everything else, you abstain from teas, from fruit juice, etc. In fruit diets (peaches, oranges, and things like that), there's a big difference, even if you're taking only fruits. When I speak about fasting, that means only taking water, no teas, no fruits, nothing else. And there's a big difference. You can get resettled by going on a two-week "cure" as they say, eating grapes or oranges or whatever. It's not a fast and it does not give the same results, under the same principles, as fasting taking only water.

I myself joined the Vegetarian Society in 1931 - even from the start I joined the sports team for young boys and girls in Sweden. The leaders were vegetarians and they spoke about it, and they had newspapers which talked about vegetarians. I took them home to my mother and said "I want to be a vegetarian." And she said: "Well, fine, let me know what to give you." I never liked meat or fish at all, and I remember when I was told to have milk, I asked my mother to put in 50% water in the milk. So becoming vegetarian for me was not difficult, and I must stress the importance of fresh raw food. Since the start, I've been eating a minimum of 50% of raw fresh vegetables or fruits.

Vegetarianism in Europe includes many who consume milk products, and some who eat eggs; they are call lacto-vegetarians and lacto-ovo vegetarians. There are people who call themselves "fish-vegetarians" - I don't know what that means - and I'm waiting to hear the word "meat-vegetarians." That means that they are vegetarians but eat some meat. The word "vegetarian" comes from the Latin word "vegetus" which means to grow and be strong, so actually to begin with it doesn't have much to do with vegetables.

Whether you're a vegetarian or a meat eater, it is very important to eat the salads - when you start a meal you should have a fresh raw salad first. You should not have it in the middle of the meal, and have potatoes or rice first, but you should eat the fresh raw vegetables first. Because when you eat the fresh raw vegetables, an enzyme is produced in the saliva, and then the enzyme acts in the digestive process all through the body. If you start with a potato or a sandwich or whatever and take fresh salad after that, this enzyme will not be produced in the saliva, as it has been shown clinically (by tests of the blood and so forth).

When you go on a fast, you don't have to do any preparation if you are vegetarian. You just stop eating without any preparation. But I would advise you, if you're not used to fasting to consult someone who knows about fasting and has been fasting himself. But if you can't find anyone like this, try a fast for one, two, or three days and then the next time, you can take a week or two or a month or two. What is important is that you don't have any worries. You shouldn't worry about anything. The purpose of the fast is to give the body a complete rest in body and soul. You should be comfortable, lying in bed, and should have access to fresh air and fresh water. When you water fast, you'll be thirsty and then you'll drink as much water as necessary to quench the thirst. You don't have to drink roughly two or three or four liters a day; that's totally wrong. You'll drink if you need a quarter of or half a glass to quench your thirst. If you need more, you drink more. When you're exhausted, the next time you'll drink will be when you need to. This is because an excess of water irritates the system, and it doesn't help you. You lie in bed, and you take it easy. You can read a book or maybe a newspaper, but it's wrong indeed to do a lot of exercise during the fast. This applies if you are fasting because you want to obtain better health. If you are very healthy already, then maybe you can walk around, but not if you're sick and want to regain full health. The first days when you skip the meals, you will feel hungry when meal time comes. That's nothing to worry about. That is not hunger. That is only a nervous feeling that will disappear after a few days. Usually after the third day, you don't feel anything; you're in a complete rest.

When you are fasting, if you sleep during the daytime during the first few days, maybe you'll think you cannot sleep at night. But don't worry about that. When nighttime comes, you will sleep, if not the full night after a few days it does regulate itself, and you'll be awake during the days and will sleep at night. And even if you are not sleeping at night, the body is at rest, and the physiological process which occurs in the body when you sleep also occurs in the body during the night while you're unable to sleep.

You go on like that day after day and then you say: "When is it time to break the fast? When can I start eating again?" Of course, some people cannot fast for more than a few days, because they work or something else, but if you have the time, you can fast for two or three months. The time to break the fast actually is when you feel hunger, real hunger. And you don't feel that in the stomach; you feel it in your mouth and in your throat. That is when you should start eating. If you don't start eating when you feel this, then the fasting turns over into starvation or hunger. Fasting is beneficial for you, but hunger and starvation are very bad for you.

During the fasting, you drink water. You should not drink fruit juice. You will not quench your thirst with fruit juice, because fruit juice, firstly, should be chewed, masticated in the mouth to mix it with saliva, and secondly, fruit juice is a food and it has to be digested and assimilated in the body. But water enters into the body without being digested.

When you feel this real hunger coming, the force to eat is so strong that you cannot resist eating. You can break the fast in many ways, but there is only one or maybe two correct ways to break it. One can put lemon in a glass of water or orange or anything, but if you take a slice of orange or a piece of an apple, chew it very well. And after a couple of hours, you take another slice or another piece of the apple, and chew that very well, after two hours more you take more, bigger and bigger; it depends on how long you have been fasting. If you've been fasting for two to three days, you can take bigger pieces, but if you've been fasting for one or two months, then you've got to break the fast very gradually.

If a man aged forty-five to fifty (or a woman) has been fasting for three to four weeks, the tissues in his body have actually got about ten to fifteen years younger. If you want to keep this, you should stick to a very strict vegetarian diet, or a vegan diet - no eggs, no milk, no animal products. If you stick to that, the results will stick with you for many, many years. After sticking to this vegan diet, you'll like it. Your health has turned up to a higher level. I will show you some fasts which have been done. Dr. Shelton said he had over 40,000 people fasting under his guidance. That's a lot of experience. But before that, do you have any questions?

Question: *When it's not for illness, what do you think about healthy people fasting? How long? How often?*
Arne Wingqvist: Well, healthy people do benefit from fasting of course, because to attain full health is a lot of difficulty, especially if you eat cooked food. If you stick to raw food, fresh fruits, seeds, nuts, almonds, and fresh raw vegetables, then it's much easier to obtain the very top health. And what is "top health?" Many people would say that it's full harmony in body and soul, and harmony with your environment and with your family and friends, and that's very correct. But full harmony, if we take it in the physiological sense, means that every one of the billions of cells in your body are cleaned out as much as possible, almost at 100%, of the poisonous end-products of digestion and assimilation. There are some poisonous end-products even if you're on fresh fruits, etc., but not so much; if you eat meat and things, then there are much more. And meat does not have the properties to effectively clean out every single cell in the body.

A healthy person who wants to fast can fast whenever he likes. Many people fast one day a week, some fast on Sundays, others fast on Wednesdays, etc. Other people fast in the springtime or maybe also in the fall. And it's always beneficial to you, always. Because most of us, do overeat, so we'll give the body a physical rest.

Question: *Is there any risk from drinking too much water during the fast?*
Arne Wingqvist: You should drink to quench thirst. If you feel that after drinking half a glass of water, or one glass, you're not thirsty, then you stop. Maybe after an hour or two or four you'll get thirsty again, then you drink to quench the thirst. Because the body does not use the over consumption, it has no use for it. And one very important thing: do not take any enemas during fasting. It's not necessary. The body knows itself when it's time; it doesn't matter if you fast a day, or a week, or a month or two. Enemas irritate the system, and are not necessary.

This is a fast I'll tell you about. There on the stage you see eleven men. In 1954, from August 1 to August 17, we were fasting, taking only water for seventeen days. The first day, we walked 50 km. from Gothenberg. The second day we walked another 50 km., only taking water. We kept on like that until the tenth day. By then we had walked 500 km., maybe a little more, maybe 530 km.(about 320 miles), taking only water for ten days. In Sweden, we have daylight, it's almost daylight all day long, twenty-four hours a day in summer. Here, in Southeast Asia, it's different. This shows the reception we received: We came into Stockholm on an off and on rainy and sunny afternoon, and the police said there were over 200,000 people out on the street to welcome us. We had a six motorcycle escort ahead of us and four behind us. We were received in a big open-air theater in Stockholm, and they had never had so many visitors to the park, they had more than 5,000 people. Many of the city people, businessman and vegetarians came to greet us. I'm the third one in the picture, the one waving his hand. The man to the left is a surgeon, he took the initiative and was the leader. When we came to Stockholm after ten days, we were examined by doctors, and the doctors said, "Well, but of course before you start to eat again." The fast lasted another seven days, but we didn't walk 50 km. a day. But we could very well have done it, we could have kept on for twelve or thirteen or fourteen. On average, we lost about 9 kgs. (20 pounds) each.

I have good friends in Bangkok - as all over - and one of my best friends is the charter president of the VegBangkok Society. It started in 1992, and I've given some lectures there. One of my friends asked me one day, "Could we arrange a fasting walkathon here in Thailand?" So in 1996, on January 20th, from the middle of Thailand, about 300 km. from Bangkok, we were joined by nine or ten people from Thailand, one from Singapore, one Chinese, one American, and four Swedes. To start out, they all walked about 40 kms. a day. I didn't participate in that one, but my friend here on the left participated, at age 79 and a half, taking only water. The three other Swedish participants were my sons, aged from 23 to 30 years; they were also taking only water. The others were taking fruit juices or vegetable juices.

This lady is Sigrid De Leo, the second head of the EVU. She lives in Switzerland. We made a 1,410 kms bicycle tour in Sweden. That is the same distance as Chiang Mai to Bangkok and return, lasting from July 15th to August 2nd, nineteen days. We were eating only fresh fruits, nuts, seeds, and fresh uncooked vegetables. I did this at the age of 78, and Mrs. De Leo was 53, and there was another Swedish man also 53 years of age. The longest tour we made was 130 kms. in a day, the shortest one was 25 kms. Previously, Sigrid had been eating greens and cooked food, but she was born a vegetarian, and after this bicycle tour she's totally on raw food.

Below is another great talk given by Arne in July 1999:

Dear Friends!

Firstly, I wish to thank the organizers of this EVU Congress, and especially Mrs. Sigrid De Leo, for giving me this opportunity to speak to you about the food of the future - as well as of today - about "Living Food."

The most precious thing in life is free. We cannot buy it, we cannot give it away or sell it. It is priceless. Without it, life can be pretty miserable. I am, of course, talking about our health. It is given to us.

Normally, perfect health is our birthright. At birth, we usually have the best health we ever will have, but how do we take care of it?

We take it for granted, and we think it does not matter how we live, how we abuse our body, and we still expect to have our health. We get sick now and then, but medical doctors take care of that.

Modern man has access to thousands of medicines, treatments, and "cures" for everything, from a simple cold to AIDS and cancer. But it is hit-or-miss. Some get "cured," while others become disabled for the rest of their lives. For some people, a severe illness might end in a premature death.

We might ask ourselves, "What is perfect health?" A person who is overweight by 10-20% is not considered sick, as long as he is strong and vital, can manage his work, etc. A person who drinks alcohol and/or smokes is also considered healthy, as long as it does not go to excess. Same with people who drink twenty cups of coffee a day, and overeat three times a day, and so on. They are also considered healthy.

But real health, as I see it, and I know that most people do not agree with me, is when you are in full harmony with nature, when every single cell in your body is as pure as pure can be, when you feel strong, both physically and mentally, when you are full of initiative, and feel happy.

My life as a vegetarian started when I was twelve years old. Actually, before that age, I did not like meat or fish. Of course, I had to eat what was served at home, but my mother was worried over what to give me. One day I came home and told my parents that I had heard that one could live on only fruit and vegetables. This was in 1931. I said I wanted to try it, and my mother said it was all right. From the first day, I liked the fruit and the vegetables, and since then I have stayed away from eating killed animals' bodies - carcasses.

After some years I eliminated the milk-products, and after many years more, I left cooked and fried foods out of my diet.

Man is the only being on earth who heats his food before he eats it. No non-human beings treat their food with fire.

Nowadays my food is fresh fruits, vegetables, nuts, almonds, and seeds. And I feel very fine. I cannot find any reason to go back to cooked, adulterated food.

People say that a person cannot exist on this diet with no bread, no boiled potatoes, no pasta, no soup, no oil, no sugar, no salt - none of what people consider to be essential to get all the nourishment we need. They say that in the cold climate which we have in the North, and during our long winters, we must have warm food. Well, I do not agree.

A person who has not been living on this natural diet for some years and had his own experiences with such a diet does not understand the value of it. It does not matter what schools and what examinations people have. If they have no experience of their own, they will just not agree to such a diet.

I have been on this diet long enough to know that I can exist on it, and exist on it very well.

I say that boiled food is spoiled food, and bread food is

dead food, but sun-cooked food is un-cooked food.

I know, and all those who have tried this diet honestly for many years also know, that this diet is the diet of the future, but not only of the future; it is also the diet of today.

It has taken me about fifty to fifty-five years of vegetarian life to reach this stage. I do not expect everybody to jump on this bandwagon tomorrow. But I would advise you to give it a serious trial when you feel strong enough to leave cooked food altogether. When you have tried it for six or twelve months' time, you may judge the value of it for yourself. If you think that on such a diet you cannot achieve anything which involves heavy physical work and strong will-power, I will tell you that Sigrid De Leo, Ronald Persson, a vegan friend, and I myself, bicycled from Kiruna in the North of Sweden, above the Arctic Circle, to Stockholm, capital of Sweden, exactly two years ago. The distance was 1,410 kms. It took us nineteen days. We ate only fresh fruit, fresh vegetables, nuts, and seeds. One day we cycled 130 kms., and on the average 75 kms. a day. We were tired at night, but we could well have cycled another 10 or 20 kms. Also cycling with us were two young girls. They cycled from Kiruna to Umea, about 700 kms., and another young girl cycled from Haernoesand to Stockholm, about 600 kms. We were feeling very fine all the time, and none of us got sick.

Ross Horne, a well known Australian author in the field of health and vegetarian food, writes in his book, *Health and Survival in the 21st Century*, about raw food:

Raw Fruit:
The Natural Food of Primates
by Ross Horne

"Fruit can provide the full complement of all required nutrients in adequate quantities, remembering that the requirement for protein and fat are much lower than generally believed. Therefore, instead of being considered merely an accessory to conventional meals, fruit should be considered in its own right as a staple food. The advantages of a fruitarian diet are:

It provides complete nourishment with the minimum of extraneous substances capable of "silting" up the tissues.

It is most easily digested, minimizing the energy required for digestion (which is substantial), thereby minimizing total food (kilojoule) requirements.

It is palatable.

It is easily obtained and easily prepared.

It satisfies the appetite when a sufficient amount has been eaten - fruitarians are always lean.

Minimum but adequate protein is provided.

Minimum but adequate essential fats are provided.

Maximum energy is available from what is eaten, with only carbon dioxide and water, which are entirely non-toxic, as the by-products.

It provides the body with adequate amounts of pure water.

It results in a favorable alkaline internal state.

Favorable intestinal flora predominate in the bowel.

Non-constipation occurs.

No auto-intoxication occurs. Fruit detoxifies the body

The blood is clean and of low viscosity; there is good circulation with low blood pressure.

There is the least wear and tear and least "silting up" of all the organs and tissues.

That fruit alone can ideally sustain human health and vigor, even without drinking water, indicates that it indeed provides the basis of man's natural diet. Further substantiation of this view is that there are about forty distinct anatomical, physiological, and biological features of humans which show unquestionably that the human body is designed mainly for a fruit diet, notwithstanding the fact that, like all animals, they can survive less successfully on a wide variety of foods.

These features range from a natural fondness for sweet foods, jaw and teeth structure, salivary secretion, the length of digestive tract, the size of pancreas, stereo-color vision, and so on. In fact, in all these respects, humans are practically identical today with the other higher primates in the wild, which, whenever possible, live on fruit.

Evidence of the suitability of fruit as a staple food and not just as an accessory to the conventional diet is to be seen by observing fruitarians who live entirely on a wide variety of fresh fruit and who display lean youthful bodies, low blood pressure, clear vision, and unimpaired faculties, even with advancing years.

A well-known human peculiarity never before connected with this argument, but which provides almost conclusive evidence, is that humans, like all primates, are incapable of making Vitamin C in their bodies, whereas other animals can (excepting guinea pigs and fruit-eating bats). Basing their arguments on this fact, many authorities strongly advocate that people should take large amounts of supplementary Vitamin C to compensate for this "error of Nature," which they put down to an unfavorable mutation in our evolutionary past some millions of years ago. To prove this "unlucky mutation" argument completely wrong, and at the same time prove that man is a natural fruit eater, consider:

The only mutations which persist to become a universal feature of a species are favorable ones. Unfavorable mutations cannot possibly do so.

To become universal to an entire species, a genetic change preventing the synthesis of Vitamin C in the body must therefore have been, at the time, a favorable change.

The only possibility of such a genetic change being favorable is for the species to have been already getting more than adequate Vitamin C, and any more was undesirable.

The only source of "excess" Vitamin C in nature is a diet of raw fruit. (Only certain tropical fruits contain such high levels of Vitamin C; many fruits contain only small amounts.) Therefore, it is clear that the human diet ideally should be based mainly on fresh fruit, and that past errors which have led to widespread Vitamin C deficiencies are dietary - not genetic - errors.

A convert to fruitarianism was the Indian philosopher and statesman Mahatma Gandhi, who, after experiencing poor health throughout his youth, became a student of nature cure at the age of thirty-two. First he became a vegetarian and then a fruitarian. After six months as a fruitarian, he said (quoted from his book *The Health Guide*):

A period of six months is all too short to arrive at any definite conclusions on such a vital matter as a complete change of diet. This, however, I can say, that, during this period, I have been able to keep well where others have been attacked by disease, and my physical as well as mental powers are now greater than before. I may not be able to lift heavy loads, but I can do hard labor for a much longer time without fatigue. I can also do more mental work, and with better persistence and resoluteness. I have tried a fruit diet on many sickly people, invariably with great success. My own experience, as well as my study of the subject, has confirmed the conviction that a fruit diet is the best one for us.

Arne Wingqvist

** It was always a pleasure to be in touch with Arne Wingqvist. Though I've never met him, I corresponded with him via email many times as I was conducting this interview. I was looking forward to meeting him one day.

After the interview was finished, I worked hard to edit it and complete this book.

I didn't hear from Arne for a few months, and was told that one day he apparently was not feeling well. He decided to go to the hospital and passed away on the following day. I do not know any other details, but it is very sad.

The few people I know who knew Arne all had wonderful things to say about him.

I feel confident his interview will help many people. The information he shares is, in my opinion, excellent.

Another person I've interviewed for this book, Ruth E. Heidrich, has met Arne a few times, and I asked her to tell me something about him.

Here is what she wrote: "I first met Arne at the IVU Congress in Chiang Mai in 1998 where he exploded onto my scene. I had just finished my talk on the importance of exercise as well as a vegan diet when he jumped up, grabbed the microphone out of my hand, turned and said to the group, "Folks, you have just heard the best talk of the whole conference!" Now, how could you not love a man like that! We became fast friends after that since we both had as our mission, to promote vigorous exercise as well as a vegan diet."

Arne, you will be missed.

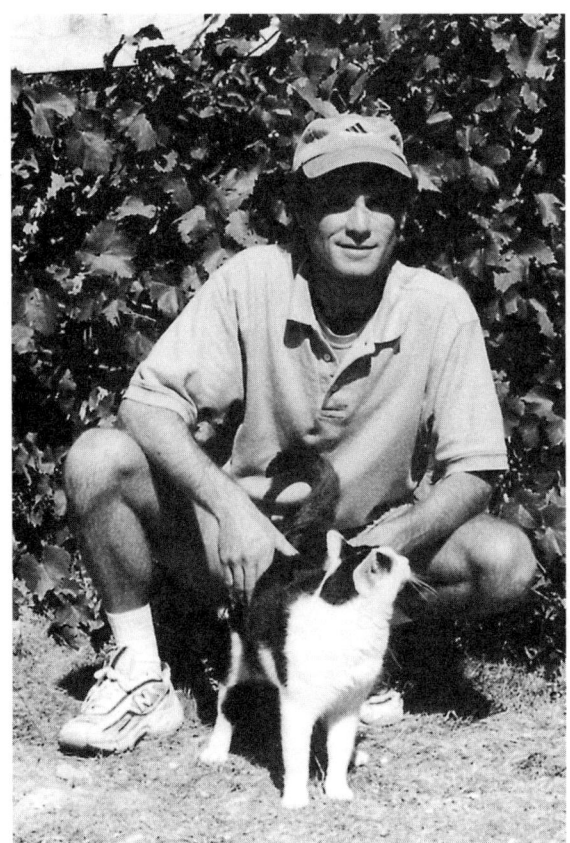
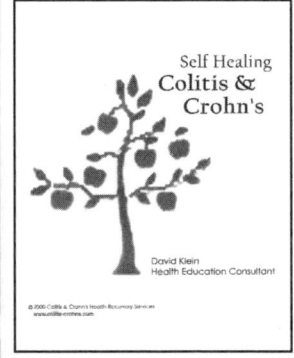
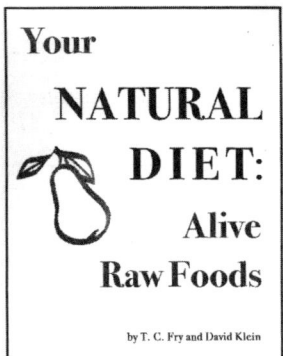

You may contact Dave at:

Living Nutrition
David Klein, Publisher/Editor
Post Box 256,
Sebastopol, CA 95473 USA
Web Site: www.livingnutrition.com
E-mail: dave@livingnutrition.com
707-829-0362

David Klein

David Klein is the Publisher/Editor of *Living Nutrition Magazine*, based in Sebastopol in northern California. David is also a Healthful Living Consultant, giving nutrition and self-healing consultations. David also directs Colitis and Crohn's Health Recovery Services at www.colitis-crohns.com

His journey from chronic illness to superb health has given him uncommon intuitive and scientific insight into nutrition and healing, through which he is able to guide his clients from illness to complete rejuvenation with consistent success. David is a living example of what he teaches and I am proud to call him a good friend.

Publications by David Klein:
The Fruits Of Healing - A Story about a Natural Healing of Ulcerative Colitis; *The Seven Essentials for Overcoming Illness and Creating Everlasting Wellness*; *Your Natural Diet: Alive Raw Foods* by T. C. Fry and David Klein; *Self Healing Colitis and Crohn's. Self Healing Power!* by T. C. Fry, Dr. Herbert M. Shelton and David Klein

How many years have you been on the raw diet?
As of spring 2002, I have been mostly raw for seventeen and one half years. I was 99% raw the first eight years, and I have been 100% raw the last nine and one half years.

How was your health when you started the diet?
My health was in unimaginable shambles after eight years of severe ulcerative colitis, from age eighteen to twenty-six. I had chronic inflammation and ulcerations in my colon, many bloody spasmodic bowel movements each day, chronic

fatigue, demineralization, nervousness, allergies, poor skin, cloudy thinking, and not much of a life. In the eighth year, my gastroenterologist recommended that I consider having my colon surgically removed. Many months earlier, I had discovered Natural Hygiene and raw food eating. It made no sense to me then, but gradually it became more and more sensible. One glorious evening, a week after the doctor's suggestion of surgery, self-healing and raw food eating all made sense. I divorced myself from medical intervention, stopped taking medicines, and plunged into a fruit-based 80% raw food diet. I healed up rapidly and discovered new joy in living. After a few months, I reduced the amount of cooked food to the point where I rarely ate it. After several years of rebuilding, with exercise, adequate rest and sleep, and other healthful lifestyle factors, I went on to experience a higher level of health than I had ever thought possible. Now I enjoy inspiring others on their path to health through my business, Colitis & Crohn's Health Recovery Services, which I direct (www.colitis-crohns.com), through my booklet, *Self Healing Colitis & Crohn's*, through the raw food lifestyle magazine I publish, *Living Nutrition* (www.livingnutrition.com.), and through the book I recently published, *Your Natural Diet: Alive Raw Foods* by T. C. Fry & David Klein.

Who are some people who have inspired you to do this?
Laurence Galant, Ph.D., a Doctor of Natural Hygiene based in Staten Island, was the health counselor who introduced me to natural hygiene and raw food eating. He gave me materials by T. C. Fry and Dr. Herbert Shelton, and they became the biggest influences in my health recovery and rejuvenation. T. C. Fry gave me great encouragement, and later on I became involved in promoting his hygiene magazine. Following his death, I began carrying on his work though *Living Nutrition*.

Is there any one person who has inspired you the most?

T. C. Fry. He had an uncanny way of presenting health sense on paper which just bowled me over with enthusiasm and set my passion for teaching others on fire. Many people have echoed this. He had a huge heart and an amazing intellect, and he was a hero to many.

You have learned so much over the years. What are some of the most important things you have learned?
I could write for hours on this subject! In my booklet *The Seven Essentials for Overcoming Illness & Creating Everlasting Wellness*, I sum up much of what I have learned about self-healing, rejuvenation, and health maintenance. Here are the seven steps: 1) Start with a healing vision. 2) Investigate, understand, and properly apply the principle of self-healing, i.e., step out of the way, rest, and allow the body to detoxify, regenerate, and rejuvenate. 3) Eat our natural biological diet: properly combined raw foods (mostly fruit). 4) Free our lives of energy-draining stress. 5) Get appropriate regular exercise. 6) Cultivate self-awareness (or mindfulness). 7) Be passionate about wellness, expressing healthful thoughts with emotion to catalyze the rejuvenation/health process.

Are there any pitfalls you have learned to watch out for on the raw diet?
Here are a few. I believe it is erroneous to place healing faith in raw food, because the laws of physiology show us that the body (not the food) does all of the healing work, acting on and using food nutrients. Food does not act on the body and heal us; our thoughts about food can heal us. Here are three other pitfalls I have learned about: 1) Eating too much dried fruit is ruinous to the teeth and unbalancing to our poise. 2) Eating too much sweet watery fruit is also unbalancing. (I eat it with neutral green foods such as cucumbers, celery, and lettuce to stay balanced.) 3) Our emotions need to be understood, honored, embraced, and, where needed, resolved, in

order for us to overcome unhealthful patterns, including emotional overeating.

Weight loss is a big pitfall for many people. Do you have any thoughts about that?
To be successful at raw food eating and be truly healthy, I firmly believe that we should study human physiology. The Natural Hygiene health science books by Dr. Herbert Shelton, the old Natural Hygiene course by T.C. Fry, and the new one by Dr. Robert Sniadach teach us how the body functions in health and disease, what detoxification weight loss is about, why and how the body will regain weight after we are cleaned out, and how the body uses food and creates energy, as well as other bodily processes and needs. People need to understand that when we eat an enzymatically active raw food diet, the nutritious, energizing sugars cause the body to spring into action, utilizing much of its energy in cleaning house: purging debris, shedding old inferior cells, and using the new raw nutrients to build a completely new, healthier body. In order to avoid the drastic cleansing that takes place when the transition is made too quickly, with its accompanying symptoms, a gradual transition is prudent.

Detoxification is a self-purifying process which the body carries out continuously, most aggressively during the early to late morning hours.

"Detox" entails: 1) the cells off-loading metabolic wastes and environmental toxins into the bloodstream for filtering by the liver and kidneys for elimination; and 2) the organs of elimination (the bowels, kidneys, lungs, skin, vagina) releasing metabolic, environmental, and residual food wastes via feces, urine, breath, sweat, and menses. Toxins are also expectorated in mucus via the throat and sinuses. The body is a magnificently designed masterpiece of self-regulation and self-healing, always striving to establish and maintain purity and wellness. There is no way around weight loss—the body needs to eliminate old stores of waste, inferior cells, and some muscle mass.

People need to slow down and take extra rest during the first few months of raw food eating, since much of the body's energy is being used to build an all-new, healthy body. In conjunction with the heightened detoxification action, the body works at repairing any damage, regenerating new cells, rejuvenating, and restoring wellness. The repair work mostly occurs when we sleep. When there is damage to be repaired and rejuvenation to be accomplished, the body needs extra sleep. We typically feel weak and need plenty of extra sleep at the beginning stage of the rejuvenation phase. If the toxemia, physical damage, degeneration, and emotional distress are severe, this phase may last for weeks or months. It is important to understand that the symptoms of the detoxification and rejuvenation process signify the workings of the awesome rejuvenative power of the body. It will help the process if we appreciate the workings of the body and do everything possible to assist it in its healing processes. We can do this by taking a break or sabbatical from our normal routines and obtain plenty of extra sleep and rest—if necessary, complete rest—and by eating simply, until the work is sufficiently accomplished and we experience new vigor and vitality. If we persevere through the uncomfortable detox symptoms and weight-loss and live healthfully, we'll be able to regain weight, build lean muscle, maintain a stronger body, and in the process, learn invaluable lessons about how the body works to create dynamic health. Remember to be patient; Rome was not built in one day.

Dental problems are another big pitfall. Do you have any thoughts about that?
Indeed. I learned the hard way. I ate too much sweet dried fruit during my first few years on the raw diet, and my already demineralized teeth suffered. I developed many cavities and ended up with many crowns. In the mid-1990s, I was fortu-

nate to meet a superb physiologist and raw foodist, Dr. Thomas Stone, a dentist specializing in full dental restoration in San Francisco. Tom teaches that during the detox phase we should monitor our saliva pH and watch for high acidity which will dissolve dental enamel. During detox, the body dumps acids into our saliva and other bodily fluids. When the pH is lower than around 6.5 (indicating acidity), we can neutralize the acid by rinsing the mouth several times per day with a watery solution of sea salt. Sea salt can be purchased in a health food store and added to a glass of water.

Tom also teaches that we can help the body replace lost dental enamel with a new mineral surface by eating mineral-rich foods and supplementing with sea algaes (such as dulse) and/or micro-algaes (such as spirulina). The minerals we digest will increase the mineral content of our saliva, which provides minerals for the surface of our teeth. I highly recommend rinsing all sea salt off of sea vegetables, because NaCl impairs metabolic functions and causes other problems. After several years, I noticed ridges developing at the top of my front teeth. After reading what T.C. Fry wrote about the mineralizing benefits of dulse in the diet, I added rinsed dulse to my diet regularly for two years. I feel that the ridges are no worse and might have filled in a bit.

I've also learned that it is very important to floss or pick one's teeth one to several times per day to keep the gums healthy.

Lastly, I believe it is wise to eat greens, celery and/or cucumber while or after eating sweet fruit to keep the teeth cleaner.

What is your opinion of mercury fillings, and what would you replace them with?
I had all eight or so of my metal fillings replaced with composites right after I went raw. My mind became a bit clearer and my jaw felt lighter after that. As the dentist forewarned, the composites developed micro cracks which led to more

cavities, necessitating crowns. Gold and porcelain crowns are the best we can do as far as I understand. Dr. Tom Stone informed me that any foreign material in the mouth can be toxic and disruptive to our natural energy field.

What is your opinion of nuts and seeds?
They are important in the diet, more so for people who live in climates where the winters are cold. However, I do not believe that we need to eat them regularly unless we are engaged in heavy exercise and want to maintain large muscle mass. The body recycles about 80% of its protein. Nuts and seeds are difficult to digest and are probably best eaten after germinating twelve hours or so in water. I love fresh walnuts, which I gather here in northern California in November and December. But they go rancid a few months after harvest. Except for almonds, which I eat once or twice per month year round, I typically eat nuts only in the winter. Avocado and durian supply more easily digested fat in my diet year round.

What is your opinion of grains?
Cooked grains were the last cooked food attachment I let go of, eight years after going mostly raw. I observed that I was eating them a few times per year simply for emotional comfort reasons. They always sedated me and caused mucus production, fatigue, and brain fog the next time I ate fruit. I experimented with sprouted grains and found them to taste bland, which leads to overeating and produces the same problems as cooked grains. I believe that they are of no benefit in the diet; all of the nutrients we need for optimum health can be obtained in raw fruit, vegetables, seeds, and nuts.

What is your opinion of fruitarianism?
Our biological, anatomical, and physiological nature, design, and disposition show that our natural diet is mostly fruit. We can say that we are naturally frugivores. I also believe that our spiritual essence shines through best on a fruit-based diet. In

practice, fruitarianism is about following our natural instincts, which I believe, after we clean out and become clear of mind and senses, will lead us to eat a diet of sweet fruits, non-sweet fruits, green leaves, celery, and some seeds and nuts when we crave fat and feel cold. A diet of 75-95% sweet fruits is generally what a person who calls himself a fruitarian eats. I believe that a diet of all sweet fruits is unbalancing and unhealthy. I feel that greens and cucumbers are very important in the diet for those who live a modern lifestyle. Perhaps those who live in the tropics and can enjoy a stress-free life can thrive exclusively on fruit. I founded the Fruitarian Worldwide Network to educate the world about how to eat fruit and to help support and connect fruit lovers. Our web site is at www.fruitariannetwork.com. My most vivacious friends eat mostly fruit, and many of us have overcome killer diseases.

What is your opinion of sprouts?
I occasionally enjoy sunflower greens and sprouted sunflower seeds in a salad. However, I don't sense a need for sprouts in my diet and find sprouting to be too tedious. I feel it is good for all raw fooders to experiment with sprouting and enjoy what feels good.

What is your opinion of Natural Hygiene?
Natural Hygiene is an organized philosophy and practice of following our senses and living naturally, in accordance with the laws of nature. Hygiene is literally the science of health. I and many others feel that studying texts and courses in Natural Hygiene provides the best educational foundation for raw food enthusiasts. My studies and my application of Natural Hygiene principles saved my life seventeen years ago. Through Natural Hygiene, we learn physiology and its application in life. Raw foodism—placing all kinds of faith in raw food and centering one's life around eating—can become delusional. Conversely, if we understand how the body works

and all of the mind/body's requisites of health, we will become more balanced and healthy than if we just focus on the food aspect. I recently co-founded the new Natural Hygiene organization, Healthful Living International. Our web site is at www.healthfullivingintl.org. We plan to rekindle the great heritage of Natural Hygiene and lead the movement through the 21st Century. We put on Raw Passion seminars, with Paul Nison and others, to teach simple raw food eating and healthful living.

What is your opinion of supplements?
I believe that the best nutritional "supplement" is a glass of fresh made organic carrot juice, or any combination of vegetable juice with fresh carrots. Powdered supplements don't come close to the benefits we receive from live juices, and they can be costly, stimulating, and delusional. However, many people are mineral deficient and need more trace minerals. They can more quickly make up mineral deficiencies using rinsed soft sea vegetables such as dulse and/or spirulina powder with vegetable salads or vegetable juices. Spirulina has given me great benefits along with rinsed dulse, although now I rarely use them. Some vegan intestinal flora products are beneficial when people with severe bowel toxemia are in the rejuvenation phase. I don't feel that they are essential or necessary on a regular basis, however.

What is your opinion of eating seasonally?
If it feels good and it is possible, then that is the way to proceed. I eat seasonal raw foods while eating some tropical or hot climate foods year round (bananas, oranges, dates, avocados), and that works great for me.

What is your opinion of fasting?
The only definition of fasting I go by is living on water and no food or juices while getting complete rest. Fasting has saved countless lives. It gives the body its best opportunity to

detoxify, heal, and rejuvenate. Our mind becomes clearest while fasting. I feel that everyone should learn about fasting properly through Dr. Shelton's books or other Natural Hygiene educators and doctors.

What is your opinion of food combining on a 100% raw diet, and is it necessary?
I believe that food combining is absolutely necessary if one has the goal of becoming clean inside and truly healthy. For people with weak or moderate digestion, it is essential in my opinion. Those with strong digestion generally do not appreciate the value of properly combining their foods. I believe that later on in life they will find that it is necessary. From what I have observed and experienced, those who eat haphazardly have, to an extent, toxic bowels and blood and clouded senses. Simple eating is unquestionably the easiest way for our digestive system and keeps us cleanest inside.

What is your opinion of physical exercise?
I believe that we all need to be active and enjoy several types of exercise. I feel that light jogging or running is very important for fitness and health, and I believe that if we do not exercise, then we don't need to eat much. Many raw fooders eat and eat and do not exercise to "earn their calories." If we eat when the body has no need for nutrients, we become toxic, sluggish, and unbalanced and we age faster than normal. Vigorous exercise feels delicious and in my opinion is essential for folks who eat.

What is your opinion of wild foods?
If they can be practically obtained, they will serve the body well. If they cannot be obtained, superior health can still be built on a diet of properly combined organic raw foods.

What do you have to say about emotions?
Understanding our emotions, our emotional nature, our emo-

tional reasons for all of our behaviors including eating, and practicing emotional awareness is vital and rewarding for raw fooders as well as anyone. Some raw food educators are now discovering this, and they are helping people with eating disorders and other unhealthful emotional patterns transform their lives. I believe that most of our eating is emotionally driven. That is not necessarily bad, but most people tend to overeat even though they are well nourished. I believe that there are two reasons why people overeat: 1) they want to cover up an uncomfortable emotion and feel something different; and 2) they feel emotionally empty and cannot tolerate the emptiness. Food brings nice feelings to the body and often helps us feel love. However, love is always present in the body. It is wonderfully liberating to avoid food and delve into the love feelings when we feel a need for food comfort. There is some new good information about emotions and emotional resolution coming to light in the professional counselor's community, and through Living Nutrition Magazine we teach emotional tools for transformation. Working at knowing our emotional selves can be very liberating, and I highly recommend working at this. I personally teach the "somatic inquiry," a meditative tool for inquiring into our appetites and learning about our true needs and deepest nature.

What are your age, height, and weight? Has your weight changed, or are there any and other changes your body has gone through? How did you handle it?
I am forty-three years old, five feet eight inches tall, and I weigh 130 pounds. I began raw eating when I was sickly with ulcerative colitis. My weight went down to 116 pounds as I detoxed, then it went up to 124 after three years. In my case, the detox symptoms were less of a problem than the illness symptoms, which of course included detox. Being so thin was mentally and emotionally difficult, but I persevered because I knew that it was the only way to regain my health and

life. In the beginning, I healed up so quickly that I was jumping with joy and thus did not let the weight loss completely bother me. I felt better, and I knew the weight loss was temporary. I am obviously not big now at 130 pounds, but I feel more energetic than ever and I have built thick leg muscles from running every day.

Did you ever get really sick or have a bad detox?
In my case, I was sick and detoxing when I began. I quickly became healthy and felt more and more youthful as the detox and nourishment proceeded. During the first year, I had brief periods of feeling down and some mild headaches, which I attributed to detox cycles. I rode them out by sleeping more, and they disappeared for good.

Do you eat 100% raw foods? If so, for how long?
Yes, I have been 100% raw since I lost all attachment to cooked food about nine years ago. It seems that remineralizing my body with some sea vegetables and spirulina helped me become 100% raw.

What is your average daily diet like? What do you eat, and how often?
I typically eat citrus for breakfast after I have gone for a short jog. I usually follow that with a few bananas or dates and either cucumbers or greens. On some mornings, I have melon. I strive to eat lightly in the morning, and I eat no earlier than 9:00 a.m. Eating breakfast after 11:00 a.m. is my goal. I then eat small meals of sweet fruits and or cucumbers three or four times per day. About one to three times per week, I have an avocado. In the summer, I have raw corn or tomato meals with cucumbers, bell peppers, and/or greens. I usually eat two heads of lettuce per day or some celery. About once every two or three weeks in the warmer months and several days a week in the winter, I have nuts with cucumbers and/or greens. About once a month, I make juicy carrot pulp in my

Champion juicer and eat it plain or with broccoli pulp.

Sometimes I mash avocado into the vegetable pulp—that makes a hearty meal! When I was rebuilding, I made fresh juices often. I rarely make juices now because it gives me too much of a sugar rush, but I'd like to get into a routine of drinking a small glass of carrot-veggie juice once per day because it feels so nourishing and it is great for my skin and hair.

What is your favorite food?
That is not easy to answer, but I'd say durian. If I have an empty stomach and am energetic and craving something sweet, a honeydew melon, fresh deglet or medjool dates, sapote, sapodilla, mamey, or durian can be ecstatic. Many fruits are delightful. If I crave something fatty, almonds, pecans, pistachios, or avocado can do it for me. If I crave something light and refreshing, salad mix or cucumbers can be exquisitely refreshing and even energizing. If I crave something salty, fresh heirloom tomatoes can make an awesome meal.

Of all foods, which do you think is the most important?
Bananas are the #1 staple food in my diet. I have eaten over 50,000 of them in the last seventeen years, and after each one, I felt great. In my opinion, they are probably the most perfect food for humans, based on nutritional content, easy utility, aesthetic appeal, availability, and economy. Cucumbers and oranges are also staples in my diet.

How are your health and energy?
Excellent, provided that I keep myself well rested. Working too much tends to drag me down, so I strive to avoid overworking and to keep myself energized and happy.

How much sleep do you get, and how much do you think is necessary?
Seven to eight hours. When I take great care of myself and eat lightly, I wake up around 4:00 - 5:00 a.m. refreshed and full of

energy on about six or seven hours of sleep. When I eat nuts or avocado, I sleep more.

What mental changes have you noticed?
Before I began raw eating, my brainpower was impaired, running at a low capacity. I was very malnourished and fatigued from a lifetime of poor eating and eight years of illness (ulcerative colitis), medications, toxicosis, and psycho-emotional trauma. I was miserable most of the time.

A few days after I began the raw fruit-based diet, my senses and mind began rejuvenating, and my spirit began to soar. My mind became clear, my memory improved and went on to be greater than ever, and my gloom was replaced by joy and vitality. I have overcome writer's block and feel far better about my whole self now.

Many people just getting into a raw diet have problems because their mates don't want to change. Do you have any comments or suggestions?
It appears to be important for partners to share common health goals and support each other, especially if they are at different levels. If one partner is unhappy with the other not changing, and if one or neither is getting his or her needs met, then counseling is usually a good avenue to take. If it becomes clear to a couple that their chemistry is not right, their goals are different, and their needs are not being met, then a conscious decision to separate might be the best thing.

Has your opinion of sex changed over the years?
Too much sex is enervating for males, even if they're raw fooders. For me, raw living is a conscious living path, offering the opportunity to look at my habits and become more mindful about sex, as well as other aspects of my lifestyle. Conscious sex, shared by lovers with clean bodies and unstimulated by meat, coffee, drugs, or power foods (including raw ones), can be an extra-special experience. I've found that my need for

sex has diminished because I feel great most of the time and don't seek the extra high as often as I used to. My libido is still strong at age forty-three, but not as high as before. That feels somewhat liberating, opening me up to feeling love even more than before.

Do you think it is harder for a woman to eat a raw diet than it is for a man? If so, why?
From what I have observed, males generally have an easier time transitioning and staying raw. I believe that females generally have a more difficult time because of their more emotional nature and because eating is such an emotional issue. Understanding one's emotional nature at a deep level and one's relationship with food and other cravings can help make the process easier. Working with a supportive counselor who understands the physio-psycho-emotional dynamics of health and raw foodism can be very helpful.

Why do you think there are more raw men than raw women?
Because of the more emotional nature of females and because our society is so stressful, creating so many issues around food and appearance. Unresolved emotional issues affect any raw fooder's progress on the path.

What are your thoughts about the female menstruation cycle? Do you think it is natural for a woman not to bleed when she is on a raw diet?
I have heard that many women's periods diminish, become lighter and, in some cases, stop either temporarily or permanently on the 100% raw food diet. This suggests to me that the cleaner the diet, the cleaner the body and the less need there is for detoxification.

I don't know why a perfectly healthy, completely detoxified female should bleed. Some people have suggested that bleeding is an adaptation due to humanity's 20,000 or so years of eating cooked food.

Do you have any comments about PMS and the raw diet?
PMS and menstrual difficulties cease after one has cleaned out and adopted a healthful eating style, not too high in acid-forming foods.

Do you have any comments about pregnancy and the raw diet?
I am not a parent, so I don't have any experience to offer. However, I have heard a few raw food mothers say that giving birth was far easier than it was when they ate cooked food.

Would you like to add anything?
Transforming our health and eating habits is a process that takes education, time, patience, self-nurturing, and support. It takes years for most people to get beyond cooked food cravings and emotional issues (it took me eight), and that is okay—we are all perfect just as we are. Raw food eating mastery is an ongoing process for everyone. I am still working on the emotional component and learning more about myself after seventeen years at it. Although I eat 100% raw foods, life has not become perfect for me; there are a lot of issues I work on every day, including overeating, overstressing, and keeping balanced.

Food is just food, and eating raw foods is just one of the many ingredients in our health recipe. Raw food provides nutrients and sensorial delight when we are hungry. But food does not heal us; our body heals when we change our thoughts and unhealthful behavior. A wise person said, "Eat to live; don't live to eat." My friend Morris Krok says, "There is no magic in raw food." As the years have gone by, I have increasingly found that consciously experiencing the joy of being with an empty stomach and a clear mind can be far more exhilarating than any raw food indulgence.

Therefore, I suggest that you enjoy your food, take a look at any fanatical behavior and judgments from within and from others, accept yourself as you are, and be good to yourself along the raw food path.

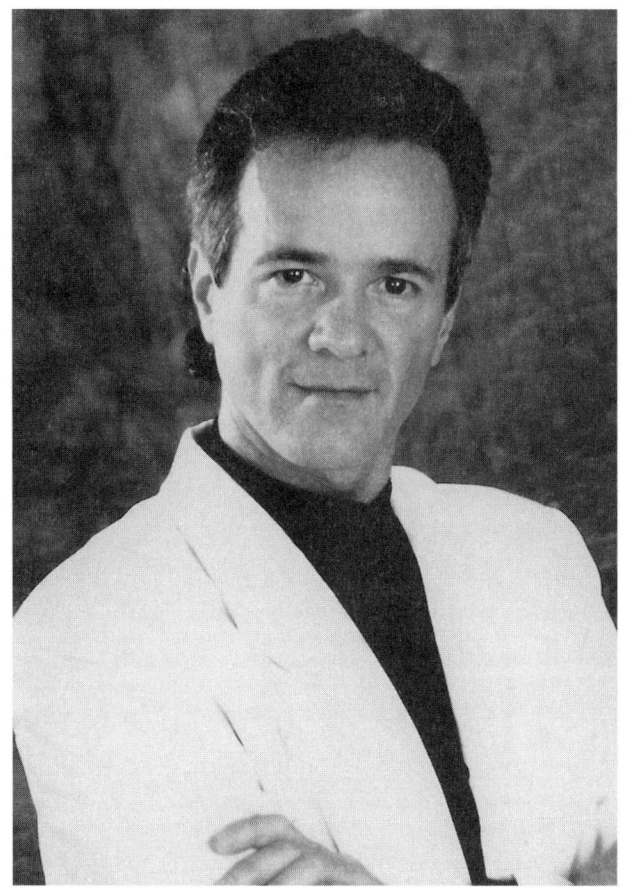

You may contact Robert at:

Dr. Robert Sniadach, D.C.
President - TRANSFORMATION INSTITUTE
School of Natural Hygiene - Independent Home Study Courses
1103 Collinwood West Drive
Austin, TX 78753
Email: rwsniadach@transformationinst.com
Website: http://www.transformationinst.com
512-835-1364

Dr. Robert Sniadach, D.C.

About Dr. Sniadach

Personal Information
Born March 3, 1957, musician, composer, mango lover.

Educational Background
Completed Life Science (Natural Hygiene) Course in 1985; earned Doctorate in Chiropractic in 1993; almost completed Bachelor of Science in Electromechanical Design Engineering previous to that; completed nine month fasting internship with Dr. William Esser in 1994. Certified member of the International Association of Hygienic Physicians since 1994; currently working on a Master's degree in "Laughing at Myself when I Get Too Serious."

Current Health Practice
Currently, runs Transformation Institute, which offers comprehensive Home Study Courses in Natural Hygiene; works directly with Healthful Living International and the Healthful Living Consultants Group (HLC), overseeing the program of student education leading to qualification for membership in the HLC.

Maintains a clinical practice specializing in fasting and detoxification programs customized for each patient. Most often works with patients suffering from chronic allergies, fatigue syndromes, and eating disorders. Conducts fasting and meditation retreats several times each year at various locations.

Fervently desires to help establish and promote the next generation of leaders in the Authentic Health and Wellness field. That is the goal of Transformation Institute.

Due to the mixing of conventional and alternative therapies around the world, there is mass confusion about health care, what "works" and what does not, what is truly health-promoting and what is temporary distraction. The continued pitiful results of traditional and alternative care and the astronomical costs that both incur have opened up the minds of a huge number of people to finally hear the pure and simple message of Natural Hygiene. Natural Hygiene is the next wave of conscious living. We are the key messengers.

Future Goals/Health Projects
The Essential Natural Hygiene Course is now available for everyone who is deeply driven to learn the truths of the natural science of good health - Natural Hygiene. For anyone who is new or relatively new to the raw/ vegan/vegetarian/healthful living world, enrolling in the Essential Natural Hygiene Course would be an excellent decision. If you are going to gather your information haphazardly over several years, as most people do, you will likely spend many hundreds if not thousands of dollars on books, tapes, videos, and so on. And though you will get lots of good information with this approach, you will also get much conflicting information, which can be very confusing. By taking the Essential Course you will save lots of time, money, and effort. All the essentials are provided for you in a logical, structured manner.

Published Works
True Health Freedom published in the Townsend Letter for Doctors (alternative care journal) and in the Somatics Journal (bodyworker journal) Natural Law - self-published healthful lifestyle magazine in early '90s.

Lecture/Seminar Topics
Many health conventions and regional gatherings on Natural Hygiene topics; Essene gatherings on the use of fasting for physical and spiritual health; many talks at various vegetarian and healthful living group meetings and churches over the years.

How many years have you been on the raw diet, and what got you into it?
I've been moving towards more and more raw foods for many years. I was probably about 70% raw ten years ago; I'm now 95% or more.

I've been studying and practicing Natural Hygiene since 1982. Personal illness (chronic sinusitis) led me through the usual haphazard, painful route: medical treatments, then alternative medicine treatments... Then Natural Hygiene popped up in my life in 1982, and my whole world has been radically changed ever since. It has been an awesome journey. Not only did my physical health improve tremendously, my mental sharpness also improved, my emotional balance improved greatly, and, most wonderfully of all, my spiritual growth has skyrocketed. It is so incredible how peaceful, blissful, and connected I can feel, and it all comes so naturally and easily with Natural Hygiene. Live and learn the Truth, and the Truth shall set you Free!

Who are some people who have inspired you to do this?
It has been a gradual process of adding more and more healthful living education to my lifestyle over the years. The most significant beacons of light have been Herbert Shelton, T.C. Fry, J. H. Tilden, William Esser and Virginia Vetrano - all Natural Hygiene writers. Others have added bits and pieces, but these were by far my main influences. Also, I have had my spiritual life enhanced by several authors in this realm - most importantly Edmond Bordeaux Szekely, who wrote a great amount of material about the Essenes and their practices. Strangely enough, very few spiritual authors have made the connection between living foods and spiritual aspirations. I hope to remedy that with the "Human Potential and Natural Hygiene" course that I will offer through my school, Transformation Institute. http://www.transformationinst.com

Has any one person inspired you the most?
That would be Herbert Shelton. He had such fire and drive behind him to get the message of superior health out to everyone. He was definitely ahead of his time.

You have learned so much over the years. What are a few of the most important things you have learned?
It is most important to cultivate the direct, personal awareness that your body and mind are a direct extension of Source/God. Every one of us is infused with Life Essence, the very same energy that drives all and everything in the universe. That being so, it is important to know that there is infinite wisdom and intelligence at work in you; an intelligence that you can trust implicitly; an intelligence that will faithfully supply you with maximum well-being in body, mind and soul; an intelligence that strives to eliminate burdens and provide disease-free superlative health every moment that you are alive... as long as you provide your body with the essentials of Life that it needs to create health. These essentials are most beautifully and profoundly presented and examined in Natural Hygiene.

All particular practices and principles flow naturally from this wisdom. It is simply a matter of becoming aware of the immensely powerful and life-giving forces at work in Nature, and allowing yourself to actively and purposefully harmonize with them. The key is in "allowing" this beautiful wisdom into your depths of Being. It is far better to allow it in, rather than to "study hard" and force it in. By forcing it becomes merely an intellectual exercise. By allowing it in it becomes a simple revelation of Truth for you, and the practice of it in daily life becomes far easier.

Are there any pitfalls that you have learned to watch out for on the raw diet?
For most people I've found that it is necessary to go gradually,

so as to maintain the best balance for one's particular situation in life. You should gradually work toward your goals of 100% healthy, living as best as you are able to. Still, some people will want to go right to the goal. All approaches are good. For many people, due to a lifetime of an extremely poor diet and lifestyle, it will take the body many months or even several years to fully regain optimal function, strength, and vigor. There are ways to accelerate this recovery of 100% health, and the most fundamental aspect is to get a firm and solid re-education in the philosophy, principles, and practices of Natural Hygiene and healthy living. It requires a large degree of internal re-programming, since most of us are filled to the brim with wrong information. By putting forth the noble effort of re-learning HOW TO LIVE, your rewards will be greater than you can imagine. As one's intellect is reprogrammed, it is also important to initiate a supervised fast for oneself. This will result in profound detoxification of all levels of one's Being, and the acceleration toward the goal of JOYFUL LIVING skyrockets.

Weight loss is a big pitfall for many people. Any thoughts about that?
It will improve over time as the digestive strength and vigor improves. It may take many months or years, as I mentioned previously. There is usually no need to worry about it. The best approach is to increase vigorous activity and exercise in one's lifestyle. This will create dramatic improvements in all areas of wellbeing.

Dental problems are another big pitfall. Any thoughts?
Be careful with overeating on acidic foods - citrus, pineapple, etc. Be sure to include plenty of green leafy vegetables in your diet, as well as other types of vegetables, preferably on a daily basis. These will help to provide all necessary nutrients.

What is your opinion of mercury fillings, and what

would you replace them with?
At this time, for filling cavities I recommend porcelain composites. There may be better state-of-the-art materials currently available of which I am not aware. I suggest that anyone who has mercury fillings should get them removed safely and refill the cavities with the healthiest and strongest composite material available. It may take some research to find the right dentist and the right materials, but it is worth the effort.

What is your opinion of nuts and seeds?
They are excellent foods. Get them raw and fresh as possible. In the shell is best. Soaking overnight is great. It activates the dormant life within; the germination process literally sprouts forth. It makes them much easier to digest as well, for the enzyme inhibitors that are naturally-occurring are then deactivated and copious nutrients are released for your digestion.

What is your opinion of grains?
They are unnecessary and damaging in the long run, but they may be useful for the newly-aspiring raw foodist to use for a while. It is best to eliminate them as soon as possible for maximum health.

What is your opinion of Fruitarianism?
Fruits should be our primary foods, but I don't recommend a purely fruit diet. Complement them with veggies, seeds, and nuts, and health will be yours.

What is your opinion of sprouts?
Several types of sprouts are good foods and make a good addition to salads. Go with the milder sprouts, not the bitter, sharp, or pungent ones. Sprouts are so brimming with Life Force that they can greatly help to revitalize and rejuvenate if health is at a low ebb.

What is your opinion of Natural Hygiene?
The KING OF LIFESTYLES! The only way to go!

What is your opinion of supplements?
Some of the higher quality green food concentrates (spirulina, chlorella, sea vegetables, etc.) can be useful for those just beginning their healthy lifestyle transitions. Most conventional diet people are malnourished in some manner, and their digestive capability is shot. As digestion gradually improves on a healthy diet, the green food concentrates can assist in the early stages. Eventually, they will not be necessary.

What is your opinion of eating seasonally?
It's an excellent thing to do as much as possible. It helps people to harmonize with their local environment and to assimilate the energies of their surroundings. Ideally, human beings should be living in climates that are warm and fruit-bearing all year round, which would provide us with our fresh, natural diet all year long. That is paradise!

What is your opinion of fasting?
Fasting is extremely useful and beneficial for those desiring to recover from nearly all types of disease. Once health is recovered, it is also very beneficial as a way to rest and rejuvenate one's whole Being (body, mind, and soul). All facets of our Being respond positively in the most remarkable ways as one wisely fasts to regain and improve health. All energies of all the Levels of our Self come together gradually, perfectly, and harmoniously as the fasting process proceeds. It is Nature's way of health recovery and maintenance.

What is your opinion of food combining on a 100% raw diet, and is it necessary?
Food combining is always helpful to the body, because it makes digestion easy and thorough. It is also wise to make a number of your meals mono-meals; that is, one food per meal, eating as much as you want until you are naturally satiated - full. This will give rise to maximum digestion and maximum nutrient assimilation. This is the way nearly all animals eat in

the wild, and it is wise for us to learn from that. Simple meals and varied diet is the key. Also, of course, ALWAYS go for the highest quality food that you can find. It is worth it.

What is your opinion of physical exercise?
Mandatory. It should be varied in as many aspects as possible. Exercise outside whenever possible to get fresh air and sunlight over all of your body. You may engage in a specific exercise one day and another type of exercise the next day. Just as in diet, keep any given exercise simple, but incorporate great exercise variety over a period of days. Strength, endurance, flexibility, speed, grace, flowing movement, focused movement, stamina are all important and healthful.

What is your opinion of wild foods?
Whenever possible – they're great! Learn about your local environment and sample the bounty! You'll be amazed at what you can find.

Would you like to suggest any other topics that are healthy and helpful?
Factors just as important as raw food are raw sunlight, raw fresh air and water, plenty of raw sleep, rawsome relationships, raw creativity, raw emotions, raw expression, raw radical honesty with oneself and others... and on and on. This is what Natural Hygiene is all about. 'Tis the Spiritual Lifestyle of Champions.

What are your age, height, and weight? Has your weight changed, or has your body has gone through any other changes? How did you handle it?
I'm currently forty-four years of age, five feet nine inches tall (175 cm), and 140 pounds (63.5 Kg). I have been at this weight ever since I adopted Natural Hygiene as my lifestyle. I was up to twenty pounds overweight before that. The pounds came off effortlessly and I stabilized at my current weight eas-

ily. It has all been rather easy for me. I initially dropped below my current weight for several months when I first adopted the program as my body broke down unhealthy tissues and structures, making way for building improved and healthier cells and tissues.

Most people will go through an "underweight" period as their bodies eliminate sickly and poorly functioning cells. They will be underweight for several months in most cases. If they stay with the program, new healthier cells and tissues will be created, and their weight will naturally increase. It will stabilize at exactly the weight each particular body wants to have. And they will feel ecstatic!

Do you eat 100% raw foods, and if so, for how long? If not, how much cooked food do you eat, and why?
I eat about 95-100% raw foods. I find that I have very little, if any, cravings for cooked foods. If I do eat them, it is mostly for taste variety now and then. I do notice that they have a subtle "slowing down and clogging up" effect, though. But as I say, I don't "beat myself up" over it. I just go with the flow of however life shows up in the moment. Personally, I also find that the warm months of the year are especially easy for eating 100% raw foods. That is the case for everyone I have ever asked about it. It just goes to show that the tropics is where we are meant to be!

What is your average daily diet like? What do you eat, and how often?
Typically, I don't eat anything for the first five to six hours that I am awake. Then I have fruit for my meals until evening, when I have a huge salad with nuts or seeds, or avocado. In the past, I tended to pick at fruits all during the day. Now it has gravitated toward specific meals with no eating in between. I'm simply following what my body tells me to do. It's much easier that way. However, it may take years for people to get to the

point where they trust their bodies' messages enough to heed them. It is very easy to get wrong messages early on in the transition to this lifestyle. There have been so many years of less-than-ideal living and eating, that the seemingly "intuitive" messages from within are all perverted from normal.

What is your favorite food?
Wow! There are so many! Truly, for me, any fruit that is perfectly ripe and well-grown is like biting into Heaven, the tropical fruits, especially. Perfect mangoes can be orgasmic. Perfect durians literally put me in an altered state of consciousness. My meditations are incredible about an hour after eating a durian. An excellent nectarine is awesome. Sweet watermelon on a hot summer day is paradise. How can I compare? They are all just perfect.

Of all foods, which do you think is the most important?
The most important things are simple meals and thoroughly chewing and enjoying the one or two to three foods you are eating. You can get great variety over the course of several days as you look at all of the several days' worth of meals all together. This way, you are easily covering all of the bases while thoroughly enjoying and savoring each meal. Again, also, I would strongly emphasize that quality foods, quality air, quality water, quality sunshine, quality sleep and so on make a huge difference between success and failure with the raw lifestyle.

How are your health and energy?
Excellent! They have literally never been better. I can truly say that my health seems to be balanced so well now that it is very easy to maintain. It is all so natural and easy to do once you have gotten to the point of your potential. Of course, there is always some fine-tuning that can be attended to, but that, too, is easy. I can listen internally to my needs and meet them simply and smoothly, as Nature and God intended it to be.

How much sleep do you get, and how much do you think is necessary?
I require seven and a half to eight hours sleep a night to feel adequately rejuvenated.

Have you noticed any mental changes on the raw diet?
My intellectual capacity has greatly increased, in that creative intelligence flows through me unimpeded. My memory is enhanced, and subtle intuitive perception is greatly increased as well. Though these capabilities seemed extraordinary to me when I first noticed them, they feel quite natural to me now. I presume that this "enhanced" mental functioning is simply the way it was supposed to be all along; I was suppressing these natural abilities due to my poor living habits early in my life.

When it comes to relationships, many people just beginning a raw diet have problems because their mates do not want to change. Do you have any comments or suggestions?
Be loving, kind and gentle... but firm in your convictions. It is YOUR LIFE we are talking about. When the Divine spark gets lit up inside you, it is mandatory that you follow its callings. The rewards of doing so are far beyond your comprehension... literally. I have experienced it myself countless times. My partners have all benefited greatly from my lifestyle as they have adapted themselves to it. I have never forced anything on anyone, but certainly it is important to teach lovingly and gradually by word and example. And even if your partner does not want to join you, these things can usually be worked out somehow, as long as both partners make room for each other. If there continues to be extraordinary friction over these matters, then it is time to look deeper into the underlying emotional patterns at work. I can guarantee you that simply eating different foods is not a life-and-death issue in a relationship. If things do get that out of hand, then either

compromise on your part is in order (not recommended whatsoever), or else separate paths may need to be taken. Every situation is unique, and can only truthfully be worked out moment by moment.

Has your opinion towards sex changed over the years?
Yes, greatly. For me, sexual relations have evolved into being sacred acts. Sometimes for me there is spontaneous celibacy happening; no desire for physical sexual activity at all. Other times, deep intimacy with another can flow effortlessly into mating/merging. There is so much more going on with intimacy than I was aware of in earlier years. This has all happened due to my own personal spiritual awakening. The union that takes place between two completely heart-opened people is ecstatic beyond anything imaginable. It is the ultimate union of two souls, in my opinion. And yet it is just another activity in the flow of Divine consciousness. If you are solidly in that flow of present moment consciousness, ALL activities are ecstatic beyond comprehension... and they are just a part of life, too. Do you follow what I mean? Everything becomes divine; nothing is more important or "better" than the rest. So there is no reason whatsoever to elevate sexual relations into some "higher" mystical practice. It is all part of Leela - the Divine Play of consciousness. Simply open yourself more to every moment of life, and the richness will be seen and felt spontaneously.

Do you think it is harder for a man to eat a raw diet than it is for a woman?
No. We are all human! If there is a problem with the diet, it is because of ego madness (habits, conditioning, emotional attachments, etc.) and misinformation, not gender differences.

Why do you think there are more raw men than raw women?
Women are compassionate nurturers by nature. The Divine

Feminine is the creator and sustainer of life. In order to nurture and care for others, it is probably easier for women not to put such emphasis on being "hard-core 100% raw." Women tend to be much more attuned to their feelings and to the feelings of others, and so they can flow with those feelings more spontaneously in the moment. If a particular moment seems to require a compromise concerning a particular food eaten at a meal, for whatever reason, then compromising is no big deal to a woman. It comes naturally.

On the other hand, Divine Masculine energy is very pointed, directed, and focused on creating and manifesting things and seeing them through to completion, making whatever changes that are necessary, and sticking to those changes. After that, there may be a natural desire to maintain their changes and perpetuate their creations... to "see it through." Therefore, men tend to be "hard-core" in their attitudes about things, especially lifestyle attitudes that they feel are an intrinsic part of their being and who they are. Men can find it challenging to compromise these lifestyle attitudes that define themselves, no matter what the situation.

Of course, balance is always the key. Each of us finds where our ideal balance point is each day, and our sense of that point gets more and more refined as each day passes. In my opinion, you should always stick with what works for you. Be kind and sincere in your actions and the requests you make of other people, and your goodness will spread like wildfire.

What are your thoughts about the female menstruation cycle? Do you think it is natural for a woman not to bleed when she is on a raw diet?
It will likely diminish considerably over time. It may even seem to stop, though that is rarely the actual case. What happens is that the normal cycling occurs, but it is no longer accompanied by so much loss of blood. Only the normal small amount of epidermal tissue sloughs off, and that may not even

be noticed, fooling one into thinking that it has stopped.

Any comments about PMS and the Raw Diet?
It should greatly diminish and eventually cease. That is what I have seen happen with women over the years.

Any comments about pregnancy and the raw diet?
The healthier and better prepared the mother is before getting pregnant, the better it is for the whole progression of the pregnancy, in all ways. There is much to say about this, far more than I can include here. Suffice it to say that all phases of the pregnancy will be greatly improved, becoming naturally easy throughout. Everything from initial fertility through a benign labor, on to easy nursing and joy throughout.

One important point I would like to make is that fertility can be greatly increased by purifying oneself with a thoroughgoing supervised water fast. I see that there are literally millions of women experiencing infertility, and this is due to atrocious lifestyles and self-poisoning with garbage foods, among other things. Rather than spending insane amounts of time, effort, anxiety and money to correct such problems with medical therapies, it is far wiser and easier to simply correct the true underlying problem, toxicosis (internal poisoning), and fertility will naturally reappear.

Do you think it is harder to be a raw fooder today than it was years ago?
It is much easier today, due to the wide variety of foods available. Were one to have attempted a raw diet many years ago, it would have required following the sun, traveling to warmth and ripe foods as necessary. That's not such a bad idea today, actually!

Where do you see the raw food movement heading in the future?
If we can keep up our enthusiasm, we can turn our beloved

planet back into the paradise that it was meant to be. Of course there will be intense, antagonizing opposition from people who cannot, at the moment, see the vision of what is possible through living naturally and living consciously. It is up to each of us to use our inborn talents to awaken our brothers and sisters as soon as possible. Even those appearing "craziest" to us are merely suffering from misinformation and a lack of Love.

We are indeed in a situation where living naturally and consciously is considered abnormal, when in fact the truth is that the vast majority of human beings are quite insane. They just tell each other that they are "normal," and so carry on in their insanity. It wouldn't be so bad if there were only a million or so people on the planet acting insanely. But now that the madness is threatening our very survival, not to mention the survival of countless other life forms, it is time for drastic action. The Natural Hygiene/Raw Food movement is the sanest, most loving, and naturally uplifting approach to life that I have experienced. My internal joy naturally and spontaneously demands that I spread the word to everyone who is ready to hear.

Thank you for this interview. In closing, is there anything else you would like to add?
I live with the conviction that all that is happening in our world right now is perfect... perfect for our continual evolution and enlightenment as individuals and as a species. The happiness that we each experience, when it fades away, leads us deeper into uncovering why it is that the happiness fades, and this leads us into seeking that which is eternal, not fleeting and temporary. And of course, our sad and lonely moments naturally lead us to seek that which is really, truly fulfilling in this earthly life. Re-learning to live peacefully and harmoniously with your body and your mind will immediately and automatically spill over into a blossoming of your innate

Spirit, a flowering that will blow open the dormant potentials that lie inside you – potentials that have been awaiting your awakening for a long, long time – potentials that cry out for expression, now! So let's do it! Together!

All the best to everyone,

Dr. Robert Sniadach
President, Transformation Institute
http://www.transformationinst.com

TRANSFORMATION INSTITUTE School of Natural Hygiene
Home Study Courses in Natural Personal Health Care.
Powerful Courses for Powerful, Motivated Students.
The Essential Course. All the Fundamentals of Natural Hygiene Philosophy, Principles and Practices. Apply your Knowledge immediately to your life. Incredibly improve every facet of it!
The Professional Program: Six different Advanced Courses will equip you for a Professional Career in Natural Hygiene Counseling, Teaching, Creating Workshops, Seminars, and more.

See our website at http://www.transformationinst.com for the latest info on the New Natural Hygiene Home Study Courses.

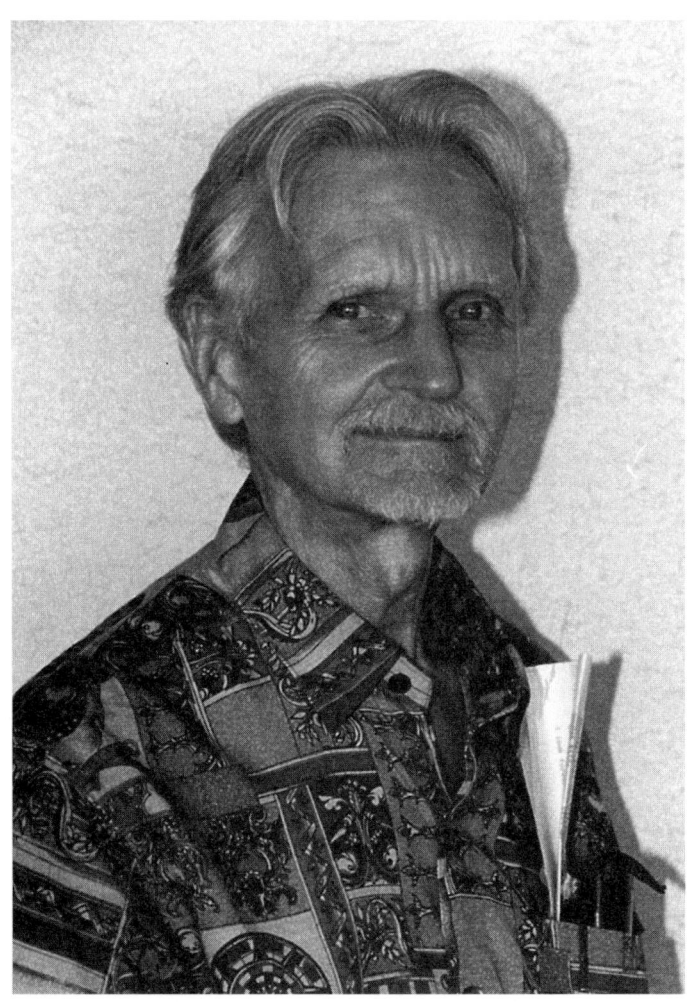

You may contact John at:

E-mail: cns03360@iig.com.au
Website: www.iig.com.au/anl/fielder.html

John Fielder

John Fielder has so much knowledge to share that I'm so glad I was able to get this interview with him. Now, just by reading it, you can learn from one of the great ones. Also, when you finish, please make sure you check out John's website for further vital information.

John Fielder's long experience in the "health through raw food" movement began before most people today were born. His credentials speak for themselves.

Below is John's bio. As you can see, he's gained much knowledge over the years.

1959 - Commenced studies in osteopathy, chiropractic and naturopathy at the Naturopathic College of South Australia, Inc.

1961 - Commenced extracurricular studies in Nature Cure under the personal direction of Kenneth S. Jaffrey.

1962 - Commenced extracurricular studies in the following disciplines:

Nature Cure, under the personal direction of C. Leslie Thomson of the Edinburgh Clinic, Scotland.

Biogenic living, under the personal direction of Professor Dr. E. B. Szekely of Rancho La Puerta, Mexico.

Natural Hygiene, under the personal direction of Dr. Herbert M. Shelton, of Shelton's Health School, U.S.A.

1963 - Was graduated in osteopathy, chiropractic and naturopathy from the Naturopathic College of South Australia, Inc.

1964 - Trained in various clinics specializing in physiotherapy, chiropractic, osteopathy, and naturopathy in and around Adelaide. Commenced part-time private practice.

1965 - Interned at Hopewood Health Centre, Wallacia, NSW. Commenced full-time private practice.

1967-'68 - Relocated to Cairns, Queensland. Established Crystal Cascades Natural Health Centre for in-patients. Established Crystal Cascades Natural Health Centre for clinical practice.

1970 - Completed extracurricular studies in Natural Hygiene, Nature Cure, and Biogenic Living. Became a member of the British Register of Naturopaths. Relocated to Clohesy River, Queensland. Established Clohesy River Health Farm.

1993 - Established Academy of Natural Living for the promulgation of the disciplines of Natural Hygiene, Nature Cure, and Biogenic Living.

1997 - Developed and presented the Natural Health Show on local radio.

How long have you been eating a raw food diet, and what got you into it?
I have been on a mostly (95%) raw diet for close to forty years and 100% for twenty-five years. I commenced to experiment with raw food due to my own ill health. Prior to commencing on the diet, I had experienced twenty-eight years of ill health. My symptoms were those of bronchitis that then developed into asthma, recurring migraine headaches, and arthritis.

Who are some people who have inspired you to eat living foods?
When I look back on things, my first inspiration was organic farming. At about fourteen years of age, I heard about the work of Sir Albert Howard, the founder of organic farming and gardening, and I read all of his books and any others I could lay my hands on. He, along with Lady Eve Balfour and Sir Robert McCarrison, founded the Soil Association in the UK, a body which is still operative and promotes, of course, the principles they espoused. They, along with two practical farmers, Friend Sykes and Newman Turner, were amongst my earliest inspirations. In fact, after studying their works, I found it hard to realize that anyone could fail to see the validity of their findings and continue to farm the orthodox way. This was long before I linked any of this to my own health problems. Why I didn't, I don't know. It was not until another fourteen years had passed that the penny dropped.

The people who inspired me once I made that link to my own health problems were, and I think of them in this order (not in order of preference, but in the order I met them): Martin Pretorius, an itinerant South African lecturer, Kenneth S. Jaffery, an Australian Naturopath, Professor Dr. Edmond Szekely, who owned a health retreat in Mexico and author of many books, particularly on the Essenes and pre-Columbian civilization in the Americas, Dr. Herbert M. Shelton of San Antonio, Texas, James C. & C. Leslie Thomson, Edinburgh, Scotland, the early writers of Nature Cure (not naturopaths), the early writers of Natural Hygiene, and Dr. Weston A. Price, and Dr. Francis Pottrenger, Jr.

Has any one person inspired you the most over the years?
Each one of these people has given me great inspiration in his or her own way. It would be almost impossible to say who has inspired me the most. I am most grateful to them all.

You have learned so much over the years. What are some of the most important things you have learned?
Everything appears to be important in its own right. Perhaps what stands out more than anything is the understanding that "scientific fact" is no truer than any other "fact." It is all based upon a hypothesis. Today's "scientific facts" become tomorrow's errors.

Are there any pitfalls you have learned to watch out for on the raw diet?
The pitfall to look out for when you are on a raw diet, or for that matter any regime, is not to listen to what our "well meaning" friends and relatives say or tell us. We should listen only to our own intuition, our own inner voice. In other words, listen to what "our" body is telling us with respect to what to eat and our other needs such as fresh air, sunshine, peace and quiet, etc. We call it "listening to the voice of the organism." It only applies to things that are natural. These things include whole raw natural food, not cooked food and/or junk food. It does not apply to unnatural substances, things of addiction, or poisons and such.

Losing too much weight is a common pitfall among people on a raw food diet. Do you have any thoughts about that?
Weight loss is normal at the commencement and may well extend over a comparatively long period of time, say six to twelve months, according to the prevailing circumstances. It is normal to go to a minimal weight and then build slowly back to what we should be. This is usually seven to fourteen pounds less than the weight/height tables on average.

Problems with teeth are also a common pitfall. Do you have any thoughts about that?
The problem with teeth appears to result from eating inappropriate foods for the climatic conditions under which we

live. This may include eating citrus fruits in a climate in which they do not naturally occur and cannot ripen. Another cause is the eating of fruits when they are not normally available. Basically you could say that I believe we should eat those foods that are natural to the climatic conditions under which we find ourselves, in their whole raw natural state.

There are many people who will think that eating perfectly is not easy to do. What do you say to that?
I am aware that this will cause a lot of people a lot of heartache. We all tend to be "idealists," myself included. What appears to me to be most important is what is "really" happening, not what I think is happening according to my "ideal." In other words, it is my belief that we must become, in the words of Buckminster Fuller, "Honest and truthful, if we are to save this spaceship earth and the life that exists upon it." Yours and mine included.

What is your opinion of mercury fillings?
Mercury fillings can be, and often are, highly dangerous, undermining the health of those who have them. There are tests that can show if they are leaching, and if they are, I would advise their removal. For myself, I would not replace them. I feel there has been insufficient research to show whether the replacements available may not be more harmful in the long term. It would appear, though, that porcelain might be the best replacement. In other words, I don't know what I would replace them with.

What is your opinion of nuts and seeds?
I believe that nuts and seeds can be a very beneficial item in the diet, providing essential protein factors. My personal experience is that in small amounts, say three to four ounces a day, they are readily utilized.

What is your opinion of grains?

Grains are best if they are minimal in the diet and, if you live in the tropics as I do, can well be completely eliminated.

What is your opinion of sprouts?
Sprouts can be a wonderful adjunct for those living in confined spaces such as a high rise with no access to a garden.

They are also fine in the cooler months to provide a good source of fresh greens, etc.

What is your opinion of Natural Hygiene?
The basic principles of Natural Hygiene are as true today as they ever were. Naturally enough, our understanding has progressed, but the principles of the wholeness of life still prevail. We still need whole raw foods, fresh air, sunlight, adequate rest, a wholesome environment, a happy social atmosphere, etc. Let us continue by being honest and admit that Dr. Shelton was not a vegan, nor were any of the earlier Hygienists. Furthermore, the principles upon which veganism, fruitarianism, etc. have been predicated (as advocated by Hereward Carrington) have been shown to be erroneous over time.

The great apes and the gorillas are not fruit and nut eaters. They eat roots and shoots and the bark of trees. These are mainly eaten with a handful of green leaves. The chimpanzee, on the other hand, has been shown to be a meat eater. The only thing we have here which is common is that what they eat is raw.

I would say that, as far as diet is concerned, if we are following the dictates of our organism (instincto) and eating the foods that are natural to the climatic condition in their whole raw state, and not in excess of our individual needs at that particular moment in time, then we are getting pretty close to what we should be doing. In fact, we are doing the best we can under the prevailing circumstances to provide the basic needs of the organism.

What is your opinion of supplements?

In the short term, supplements often appear to be very helpful. It has been my experience that in the long term, they are decidedly harmful. They most certainly are not the same as food in its whole raw natural state. They have been processed in some way. They appear to act as stimulants. It is also possible that they overload the body with the nutrients they contain. This can constitute a form of "over-eating." There is an old saying, "A drunkard may live a long life, but a glutton never."

What is your opinion of eating seasonally?
I believe that this goes without saying. Our needs vary according to the seasons. And as I mentioned previously, if we follow the dictates of our body, choosing only whole raw foods natural to that climate it will be right for us.

What is your opinion of fasting?
As with eating, activity, rest, etc., fasting is a very important part of our lives, even if it is only from one meal to the next, as most people don't even do this.

What is your opinion of food combining?
If we will follow the dictates of our body, choosing from only whole raw foods, then we can forget food combining. It has been my experience that the body will often tell us to combine foods which go right against the food combining tables but which are correct for that moment. Try to combine the same foods tomorrow, and it might be entirely wrong, unless the body tells you to. It is only right for that moment, not for all time.

What is your opinion of physical exercise?
Physical exercise is a very important part of life and necessary for our health and well-being. I believe that we need to be physically active to the point of perspiration at least once everyday. Activity is life. Inactivity is death. When we are inactive (still and sedentary in our habits), the lymphatic system

shuts right down. The lymphatic system is as important as the circulatory system, perhaps even more so.

What is your opinion of wild foods?
Wild foods have not been denatured by man, so they can be a very beneficial adjunct to our diet, providing us with many essential and beneficial nutrients.

What diet do you recommend for domesticated pets?
I have kept dogs for many years and have always had healthy dogs. They were always fed raw meat and grated vegetables. I always made sure they were not overfed and that they had lots of exercise. At least one third of their diet should be vegetables. As with us human animals, they need fresh air, sunlight, and exercise as well as raw food to keep well. If the least we do is to add blended lettuce, I would consider that a very positive step. In the course, I have prepared a section on the keeping and care of domesticated animals.

Other than my own experience, I have contact with a number of veterinarians and dog-breeders who have also found this to be true. In fact, the veterinarians recommend that dogs which have cancer should be fed two-thirds vegetables and one-third meat. Cats should be fed two-thirds meat and one-third vegetables.

The vegetables used are those which we humans would normally eat in their raw state. (Or should I say "can," since so many people do not realize that very few, if any, of the foods that we normally cook could not be eaten raw.) I must add a warning though: rhubarb, cassava (manioc), and a number of other tropical root vegetables are highly poisonous. Except for rhubarb, the others are traditionally washed and sometimes pounded and continually washed prior to being cooked to remove these poisons. Our dogs have always eaten most of the fruits that we do. If the dogs have not been brought up with this type of food, it is sometimes necessary to mince it all up together for them.

What are your age, height, and weight?
I am seventy this year. My height is five feet six, and my weight varies from 105 to 112 pounds. In the last few years it has dropped by about seven pounds. It used to be 112 to 119 pounds, which I maintained from the time I was about thirty-six years of age. That is about thirty years. Prior to that, I was never above 126 pounds.

Have you ever had a really bad detoxification, or were you ever really sick?
During the major period of regeneration, I spent more time fasting than feasting. Over one period of about six months, I would just be getting back onto whole food after a period of fasting for three days and have to fast again. When speaking of fasting, I am referring to the drinking of water only. I would fast three days, have a day on juice, then whole fruit, then a salad. That was about as far as I would get before I would develop another headache (migraine) and have to fast again. It is well to keep in mind that I had been taking medication for the headaches and the bronchitis almost continually for as long as I could remember.

My most memorable periods of illness involved mainly things that I consider self-imposed, such as accidents. I consider them self-imposed, and I also consider the habits which caused my original illnesses to be self-imposed. The difference is that in the former, I was ignorant of the facts, although this did not absolve me from experiencing the penalty. In the latter, of course, I was aware of the causes and the effects, which I duly experienced.

One accident was poisoning from treated timber when I impaled my foot with the top of a dead tree, and another accident was when I rolled a tractor on top of myself.

One other illness was the development of a pre-cancerous

condition in my bottom jaw at the site of the only dental X-ray I had ever had, which occurred over twenty years prior to the manifestation of the condition. Commonly termed, it was a radiation burn.

What do you eat on an average day?
My average daily regimen is two meals a day. I eat the first meal around 11:30 a.m. to 12:30 p.m. and the second meal around 5:00 p.m. to 6:00 p.m.

For lunch I usually have from one to three types of whole raw fruit and some mature coconut. My evening meal is usually made up of leafy greens, tomato, cucumber, celery, and avocado, along with some nuts, seeds and dried fruit. In the summer I tend to eat more fruit, and in colder weather more salad. Also, once a week, I eat about four to six ounces of natural goat's yogurt. There are periods of time when I may not eat it for a number of weeks at a time, but at other times, I might use it up to twice a week for a few days or weeks according to what I feel my body is telling me.

What is your favorite food?
My favorite food is whatever I am eating at this moment in time. That which my body (organism) is telling me to eat.

Of all foods, do you think that one is most important?
As for my favorite food, the food that I am eating at that moment is the most important.

How are your health and energy?
I consider my health and energy to be excellent by comparison with the rest of the population. I work seven days a week; my time out consists of at least a couple of hours in the middle of each day for myself. If I don't get this for any length of time, then I find it necessary to take a few days off. I have a city clinic which I attend two and a half days per week, I run a farm, I have a course in Natural Living, and I prepare and

present five radio programs, representing seven half hours of airtime per week.

How much sleep do you get, and how much do you think is necessary?

I prefer to get eight hours of sleep per night, as I feel best when I do. I can get by on six hours of sleep, but I do not function at my best under those circumstances. For me the hours before midnight are better than those after. From my observations, it would appear that most people follow this same pattern. On the other hand, there are others who are late-nighters, preferring to go to bed late and get up late. Some people feel well on six hours of sleep. Less than six hours though, for all concerned, appears to cause sleep deprivation with a subsequent loss of proficiency and efficiency. As in many things, I do not have all the answers and can only share my experiences.

What mental changes have you noticed?

My mental clarity seems to have improved in the earlier years and remained stable for the past thirty years.

Many people just beginning a raw diet have problems because their mates do not want to change. Do you have any comments or suggestions? What are your thoughts about relationships?

At the commencement of any relationship, we all tend to play roles, and these roles can continue for a period of up to two years or more until one day, we wake up and look at our partner and discover that in spite of the fact that we have been together for that period of time, we discover that we are confronted by a total stranger. When we stop playing our roles and be our true selves, we can become that total stranger to our partner, and our partner to us.

The ideal relationship is one where both partners follow at least a similar lifestyle. When either one of the partners is living on a poor diet, smoking, drinking alcohol, or using drugs, etc., then I believe the relationship is doomed, unless that partner is willing to change.

Hopefully, one will find a partner, despite all these hurdles, who is at a somewhat matching point in his or her journey along the path of life so that together they may be able to build a successful relationship. Some do, and if they do it, then that means it is possible.

Do you think it is harder for a woman to be on a raw diet than it is for a man?
I do not think it is any harder for a woman than for a man to eat a raw diet. I have yet to see any evidence that it might be true. But then, my knowledge is limited.

Do you think there are more women or more men on a raw food diet?
I would think more women.

What are your thoughts about the female menstruation cycle? Do you think it is natural for a woman not to bleed when she is on a raw diet?
I am aware that there are many opinions on this question. My observation has been that women's menstruation returns to being in conjunction with the phases of the moon and is twenty-eight days almost precisely.

It would appear that it is not natural for women to bleed. A number of women I have known who continued to be fertile and produced healthy children have told me that all they have experienced is a slight mucus discharge, which appeared to be the ejection of the unfertilized ovum, and which they described as being like "wetting your pants."

Bleeding, or perhaps we should refer to it as hemorrhaging, only appears to occur in the toxic body, such as a nosebleed. It is the body's way of eliminating excess toxic waste.

What are your thoughts about the effects of PMS while on the raw diet?
When women experiencing PMS adopt a raw food diet, its incidence is always reduced and eventually disappears. As with all major changes in direction, a woman should not expect it to happen overnight. It may well take nine to eighteen months to be completely eliminated.

What are your thoughts about the raw food diet and pregnancy?
I have never observed any problems with a raw food diet and pregnancy, but this should be noted by all mothers: STOP – LOOK – LISTEN! Do not change your diet just prior to or during pregnancy to a raw food diet, or any other diet for that matter, unless you wish to experience problems with making your baby ill.

Thank you for this interview. Is there anything you would like to add?
As a last word, I would like to comment further on exercise. It is my considered belief that we are best off if our physical activity each day is obtained through productive work that provides for the needs of ourselves and our families. Exercise obtained this way is more fulfilling, and saves much time and prevents the unnecessary expenditure of energy, especially if this productive work can be directed to the growing of our own food and the maintenance of our dwellings, etc., as it would be if we lived in a natural state.

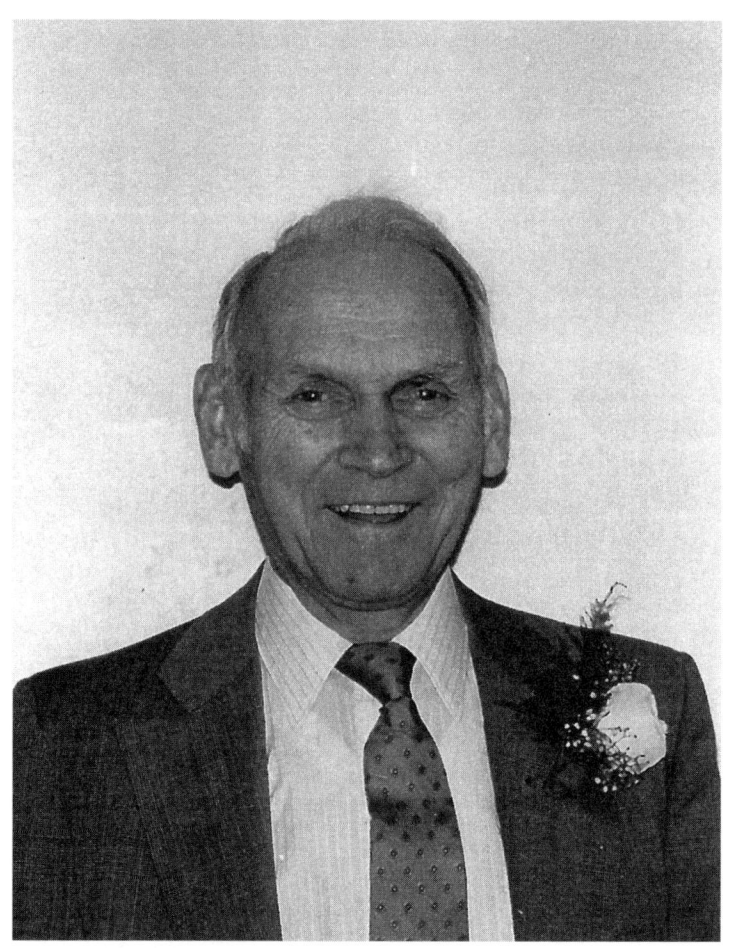

You may contact Arthur at:

Arthur Andrews
PO Box 227
Boulder Creek, CA 95006

Tel: 831-338-9416

Arthur Andrews

Arthur Andrews ran a fasting retreat in California for many years. His very close friend, Dr. Herbert Shelton, worked with him. Today, Mr. Andrews, at 80, is living life to its fullest. Many people I interview talk a great deal about food and eating when I bring up the subject of health, but in Mr. Andrew's interview, much of the information focuses not on eating, but on all the other important aspects of health: emotional control, environment, spirituality, etc. Because Arthur has worked side by side with Dr. Herbert Shelton for more than ten years, I don't think there is anyone alive who knew him better. Read all about what Arthur has learned and why he's a trail blazer in the health movement.

How many years have you been on a raw food diet, and what got you into it?
I learned about Natural Hygiene shortly after World War II. That was around 1945. I have attempted to eat a raw food diet ever since, rather unsuccessfully, or erratically, I might say. The longest period of time I have eaten purely was two years. There have been several stretches lasting two years each when I have been able to maintain absolute purity. Other periods of time have lasted six months to eight months. It has been an on and off thing.

Who are some people who have inspired you to do this?
The most important person in my life is probably Dr. Herbert Shelton. He was my mentor, my hero, my friend, and my inspiration. He is one of the really great people who have been in my life, and I have been privileged to have a lot of great people in my life - exceptional people.

You have been in the field of raw food healing for so long and with such dedication. Do you feel that your knowledge about the raw food diet and lifestyle surpasses that of most people living today?
First of all, let me make a distinction between my opinions and my knowledge. When I have knowledge, I don't have opinions. Opinions are only positions I can hold when I don't know. If I know, I know.

You have learned a lot over the years. What are a few of the most important things you have learned that might help people who are getting into this now?
Read and study books by Herbert Shelton. Don't just read his work; don't just glance through; but read and reread. The more you read Shelton, the clearer you become.

What are some common pitfalls you see people fall into when attempting this diet?
Thinking they can do it halfway. Not being willing to go to any length and go all the way. Another common pitfall would be to view it as a physical thing rather than a spiritual thing.

Many people attempting a raw food diet have trouble maintaining a weight with which they are satisfied. It is a common setback for many people. Do you have any comments about this?
Most people who got into this diet because of weight issues are very happy with the weight they lost. I have seen people go from 525 pounds down to 170 pounds and be very rapturous. There are some people who lose more weight than they would like to. For them, I would suggest that they learn that weight is not an issue. A lot of people who are into this sort of thing view it only as a diet instead of realizing that it is really a lifestyle. It is much more than a diet. It is rather a split thing. Although the raw diet is the proper diet for human beings, it's the least important aspect of Hygiene, even as it is the most

important aspect of hygiene.

What is your opinion of nuts and seeds?
They are good to eat if you happen to like them. You can overeat on them, but you can also undereat on them. It is essential to get some in your diet. If they are not available to you at all, you're in a bad place.

Do you feel that nuts and seeds are essential for protein on a vegan diet?
When I ask people what protein is, they usually start talking gibberish about what they read or heard about. The truth is that they do not know what proteins are, other than something to talk about, something we supposedly need. The truth of the matter about proteins is that practically all foods contain protein, with dates being probably the greatest exception.

Are you saying that there is no protein in dates?
I don't think so. They are not considered a significant source of protein.

Do you think someone can live healthfully without eating any nuts or seeds?
I do not consider that a desirable thing; but yes, there are people who live pretty well without seeds and nuts. I think that some nuts are useful in a balanced diet. Some seeds are useful in a balanced diet as well.

Do you think it is important to soak the nuts before you eat them?
No, I don't. There may be some people whose digestive systems have degenerated or deteriorated whose plight will be eased somewhat by soaking them beforehand.

You have to understand that nuts, as we know them, are not a raw food. They are dried food. I doubt you have ever had a raw nut. I remember the first time I had a raw almond. It was a great surprise to me. The almonds you buy in the package, Diamond almonds, are not raw; they are dried. The idea of soaking them is about as useful as soaking a dried apple, as far as doing anything favorable for it. The dried apple certainly has very little resemblance to an apple from the orchard. The latter is delicious. A slice of a whole Washington apple is one thing, and a slice of a dried apple is another. They are not the same foods. As far as nuts go, a raw almond is such an exquisite thing. No amount of soaking it will restore a dry one to what it was.

When you say that nuts are dried, are you saying they are dried naturally by the sun, or does man dry them?
It doesn't matter. They are dried; they are not a fresh food.

What is your opinion of grains? Do you consider them to be healthy?
They are useful. As far as being necessary or essential, we would probably be better off without them, depending on what we had in place of them. That is the idea: if you are not going to eat grains, what are you going to do?

Do you eat grains? If so, how do you prepare them?
Sometimes I do. Sometimes I have oatmeal. I soak it and I eat it.

Did Herbert Shelton ever consume grains, as far as you know?
At times, yes he did. For a long time, Herbert Shelton served cooked food to some people, and he did this for many years.

Did your friend Herbert Shelton live by the laws of Natural Hygiene?
Herbert Shelton lived through evolutions of his own. There was a time when he used enemas. There was a time when he realized he shouldn't, and he stopped. But that did not mean there would never be a situation where he might use an enema, even though he did not approve of them or think they were necessary; in certain isolated situations, he might think of them as necessary. He was very open-minded. Shelton him-

self did not live very hygienically. He ate well, but he did not eat very hygienically.

When I first met Shelton, he kept a barbell handy and lifted it fairly regularly. But I never knew anybody who rested less than Shelton did. Shelton used to get by on less than two or three hours of sleep a day for years and years and years. Overall, I think when Shelton was at his worst, when his nervous system was deteriorated so much that he could not hold his hands still, his skin was still like a baby's. It was soft and beautiful.

What about a fruitarian diet (living on only 100% fruits)? Do you think that is realistic?
I think that is terribly unhealthy. I have had too much experience with that myself and have observed other people who have come to me for help. I have seen the damage that can do.

We could live the rest of our lives without a single piece of fruit. We have a whole body system designed to convert starches into the sugars that we need. And if we get that out of balance, we end up with a thing called diabetes. It is called sugar diabetes. But that is not to say that fruit is bad; it is very wonderful. I would hate to be without fruit. But it is very addictive. At one time, my good friend Terry Fry (T.C. Fry) had the strongest teeth - he could crunch anything; he could even crack Brazil nuts with his teeth. I saw him lose them all, because he became a 'sugar-holic.'

Do you feel that Natural Hygienists in general indulge too much on fruit?
Yes. I don't think that the raw food diet should be more than 50% fruit, max.

How important do you think greens are?
I basically recommend to people who try it to go one-third fruit and never more than 50% fruit.

Do you think sprouts are important?

I think they are overrated, terribly so. That doesn't make them bad, but they are an incomplete food. They have not matured, and just as kids have not matured, you shouldn't put a tremendous amount of responsibility on them, because they have not had enough experience to go with it. A piece of food should be matured the same way; it benefits as it ages.

What about water consumption on a raw food diet? Many Natural Hygienists believe that you're getting enough water if you're eating raw fruits and vegetables.
I seldom take a drink of water. That doesn't make water bad. Maybe I should drink more, but I never have. If the rule is, "Drink when you are thirsty," then I almost never drink.

You mentioned dental problems for people who consume too much fruit. Are dental problems a big issue?
I do not have any teeth myself. But it's not because I ate too much fruit; it's because I ate a poor diet.

Do you feel that a lot of people on a raw diet are eating too much fruit and it is affecting their teeth?
Probably. Sugar eats away at the enamel, and it erodes.

What is your opinion on supplementation/vitamins or so-called super foods/green powders?
I don't agree with them at all. If I needed to walk to Utah every morning for breakfast, that might be something that would help me, but I am not going to walk to Utah every morning.

What about the common athlete today who wants to try a Natural Hygiene diet? Do you think it would be beneficial for him to add supplements to his diet?
If anybody wants to try something, let him try it. I am 100% for freedom.

What is your opinion of eating foods that are only in

season or locally grown?
My wonderful friend, Herbert Shelton, had a lot to say about that. He said, "Practice your hygiene wherever you are." If you are in a place where apples are growing, then you should eat apples. If you are in a place where oranges are growing, you should eat oranges. But try to get a balance in your meal. I think you are better off if you can eat the foods that the soil provides wherever you happen to be.

Do you think it is harder to eat a raw food diet in a colder climate?
Sure. Obviously, it is harder to do. If you are going to do it at all, you are going to have to depend a lot on polluting aspects of air travel and shipping foods and storage and all those things. You are better off if you have a plot of ground of your own, and grow your own.

What about the times when people eat? Do you feel that eating late at night is a problem for people?
Most people eat all the time, whenever they get the opportunity. Sometimes they create the opportunity if there isn't one. It should be a case where less is superior to more. As for the time you eat, you are probably better off going to bed on an empty stomach, or a nearly empty stomach. You should probably stop eating several hours before you go to rest.

Do you think most people today eat out of habit or for true hunger?
Most people are victims of advertising. They are victims of their own practice. We have to eat to keep the economy going. It is one big reason and it's a very serious issue. Who would go to work or who would pay the bills if you didn't have a job? And how many jobs are tied to the food chain thing? Look at all the practices; look at all the factories!

I think people would be better off if they ate less. I think people are eating especially out of boredom. But they have other things they can do with their lives that are more useful.

What is your opinion of fasting?
I like fasting. I have fasted for more than 300 days over the last ten years. My longest fast lasted thirty-one days. There have been many times when I have taken twenty-one day fasts or fourteen-day fasts. There was a period in my life when I would fast for seven days, then eat for fourteen days, then fast for three days, then eat for six days. That would comprise one month, thirty days. I would fast an extra day if the month had thirty-one days. I did that for months and months and months and exercised very heavily during that time. I've never felt better. I never had more energy, more strength, more stamina and more endurance. Fasting is an outstanding practice.

During the fasting periods, you say you were exercising vigorously?
I was doing thirty-one miles a day on a bicycle.

Some Hygienists say it is best to stay in bed and just rest during fasting.
My friend Bernard Zovluck is a Hygienist, and he says, "Get in bed, close your eyes, cut out all sound." It's almost like sensory deprivation, and the more you keep your eyes shut, the better the healing progression. And he is right. Let go of your mind. Don't think of anything either. Space out!

I know several Hygienists who say it doesn't make sense to fast one day a week. But, I know some people who've fasted one day a week for a long time. What is your opinion?
One of my early students was a young boy named Jack Welch. He was one of my better students many years ago. He said, "Mr. Andrews, every time I miss a meal, I feel that I have a victory." If you can fast one day a week, you are ahead of the game, because more than likely, you are going to eat seven days a week unless you get in one day of fasting. Anytime you

miss a meal, you are ahead of the game.

Tell us a little about your health sanctuary.
It was called The California Health Sanctuary, an adjunct of the Religious School of Natural Hygiene. My associates and I ran it for eight years in Hollister, California. We had accommodations for fourteen students and a staff of fourteen. We took care of all kinds of sick people. We didn't have any healthy people come; everybody who came was sick. We didn't get any first-timers either; we had the people whose doctors had given up on them, and they had given up on the doctors. We had people with all kinds of diseases. We also had a lot of obesity, of course. You name it, and we had it pretty much.

How successful were you in curing all these cases?
We did not deal with "cures." That is a bad word. We didn't "cure" anybody. We gave the body its optimum opportunity to heal itself; that's all. Most people did just that - they healed. We had some remarkable healings.

What is your opinion of juicing?
Some of them taste pretty good. If you can squeeze it and drink it as it comes out, that is the only thing that makes juice great. I know that juices are not proper food, but they are okay. They can be useful. We didn't put anybody on a juice diet at The Health Sanctuary, but sometimes we used juices in breaking the fast.

What is the best way to break a fast, or do you feel it varies according to the individual?
My friend, Herbert Shelton, said that you can break a fast on beefsteak if you want to. Personally, I like to break a fast on some fruit juice and some vegetable juice for about three days, increasing the amount of juice from the first day until about the third, and then starting in on some solid foods.

Do you think that proper food combining is necessary

when eating a raw food diet?
I think the ideal is the mono meal, eating one food at a meal, in modest amounts, or eating simple combinations, under conditions of non-stress and non-fatigue. That is the ideal.

How important do you think exercise is?
I think exercise is very important. I like exercise. I like to lift weights. I like to run. I like to climb rope. That is my number one thing.

What is your age?
I am seventy-eight years young.

Do you feel that the average lifespan today can be lengthened if we consume a raw food diet?
Our current lifespan is about one-tenth of what it should be. We could rebuild something much more significant than it is. People talk about 100 years being great. I will make 100, no trouble. I will invite you to my 100th birthday party right now. You reserve that date: March 19, 2023.

Hilton Hotema talks about people easily living up to 150 to 200 years. What do you think about that?
I think that is childhood. If we can make any use of Scripture, I think there is a lot of use to be made of holy writings. Men actually began to reproduce significantly when they were 130 years old. This Scripture is rather interesting. We have early records of people living to be nearly 1,000 years of age. If you follow Scripture through, you will find there is a decline in longevity, a staircase downward, where we once lived 800 years, then 700 years, then 600 years, and finally we got down to 110, and that is about where it has stuck today.

What are your height and weight? Have your height and weight changed over the years?
My heaviest weight was about 197 pounds. That was in 1945. I was in the Army at the time. Now, I weigh about 150 pounds.

I was five feet eight inches or five feet nine inches tall at one time, but now I think I have shrunk an inch. I'm not sure. I do not weigh myself, and I don't stand up and measure myself. I know I can stand tall, and I feel good. It is nice at age seventy-eight to know that I do not have an ache or a pain in my body. That's pretty good.

In your opinion or according to Natural Hygiene, what is the definition of true hunger?
It's not when your stomach grumbles. That's not hunger. It's not when you're craving something. That is not hunger. I know a lot of people who say they've been hungry, but I have gone thirty-one days without food and not been hungry. The best I can do to describe it is to compare it to thirst. I do know what thirst is. There have been times I've been thirsty, and at that point, I did not want Coca-Cola or root beer or anything like that; I just wanted water, preferably cool. When you take that first swig of water, it satisfies. Once you've had it, you're done. That's what hunger is like, only in terms of food, not in terms of liquids.

Have you ever felt true hunger?
I have only been hungry once in my life. I mean that seriously, there has been only one time in my whole life where I have been truly hungry by any Hygienic definition of hunger. It happened when I was about thirteen years old in Cleveland Heights, Ohio. It was during the summer. I had been swimming all morning, and I was coming home from the swimming pool. As I was walking home, I got to the corner where a little shopping center was. I felt a whole different thing. I really wanted something to EAT! There used to be a bakery there. It was during the Great Depression, and I had a penny. I had this tremendous urge to eat something, and I went inside this bakery, where they sold day-old rolls. For a penny, I bought a horn-shaped, poppy seed roll. I walked outside feeling like a millionaire. I ate

that poppy seed roll with no butter, no jam or anything else. It was the best-tasting thing I had ever had in my whole life. When I was done, I was satisfied, and that was the only time in my life I can remember being truly hungry.

What is your favorite fruit?
That is a variable. I play a game sometimes that goes: if I only had one type of food for the rest of my life, what would it be? It is kind of a toss-up. Oranges, watermelons, and white seedless grapes would all be high on my list.

How are your health and energy?
My strength is good. My energy is fine. I find that I take longer to recover if I exert myself. I find that at my age, it takes longer to come back to optimum than it used to. I have abused myself considerably in my life. I do not say that with any pride or anything like that; I just know it has happened. I have been considerably a workaholic. I like physical labor. One of my fun things is to move furniture. I like to do it myself. I like to take a big desk and move it upstairs by myself. I find some way to do it. I am not talking about getting a forklift. I like to do those things myself.

How much sleep do you get a night on average? How has your sleeping pattern changed as your diet has changed throughout the years?
I would say that for most of my life, I have slept less than most people. I had the most productive period of my life many years ago. I went for eighteen months on no more than four hours of sleep a night, averaging about two and a half hours a night. Sometimes I would go ninety-six hours straight without putting my head on a pillow. I did that for a long period of time. I am not advising that; I am not saying it's good. It was necessary for me at that time in my life.

Why were you sleeping so little?

To achieve a goal. I came to a point in my life after my military service, and I learned about Hygiene. I wanted to go into teaching. I had a wife and two children and I had a really good-paying job for a young man. But, I decided to go back to school. I promised myself that my change in income would not affect my family's lifestyle. I would not require them to become paupers because of my decisions. I went back to school at Washington University in St. Louis, Missouri. Because I was eating a Hygienic diet, I knew I could do some things that other people couldn't. I carried a full graduate load. Sometimes, I would carry twenty-four semester hours at a time. During that time, I slept a maximum of four hours a night, averaging two and a half hours of sleep a night for eighteen months. I was doing heavy physical labor, I ran cross-country, I was on the track team, and I coached. That was a marvelous time in my life. I really produced. I exhausted myself, too.

Do you think sleep is important?
I think that sleep is really an unnecessary thing except for the condition we are in. I think if we were in the right, proper condition, we would not need to sleep at all. There would be no need for rest. I have not had contact with or known about anyone who did without sleep except for one person. Many years ago, back in the fifties, there was this one case on record of a man who never slept in his whole life. When he was an infant, he never slept. His case was charted out scientifically for years. I guess he finally died. He never slept, ever.

Couples often have problems with their relationships when one partner decides to follow a raw path and the other doesn't. What do you recommend to people in this type of situation?
Expect the relationship to deteriorate. It is less likely that the relationship will last, in my experience. By the same token, the fact that two people are on the same diet doesn't guarantee

them successful happiness. I am told that Marilyn Diamond, the co-author of the book *Fit For Life*, left her husband Harvey for her tennis coach.

How should people new to the raw food diet deal with friends and family members who do not respect their individual choices? What is a good way to deal with social pressures?
Get over it. I don't mean get over the diet; I mean get over worrying about the friends and the social aspects. Herbert Shelton taught me this. Whenever somebody would ask why he ate rabbit food, he would say, "Better that than buzzard food."

I still remember a business dinner of some kind that I attended in St. Louis many years ago. I was just trying to carry on a conversation with the people next to me. A guy across the table from me kept looking at what I was eating. He wouldn't let it go. From the other side of the table, he asked, "How come you are eating that? You don't like meat?" All the usual questions. I finally put my fork down and I said to him, "Are you really interested in what I eat?" and he said, "Yes," and I said, "Well, let's schedule an appointment. But I am not here for this. If you are really interested, I want to tell you about this, but if you are asking just to rain on my party, don't do it." That shut him up.

Do you think it's easier for a man or easier for a woman to eat a raw diet these days?
I know I have had a hard enough time myself. Men and women definitely have different points of view in terms of their own body images. Women tend to fear fat, and men tend to welcome the fat and think of it as more manly and enhancing their masculinity. They feel they are stronger and bigger because of their excess. A couple of weeks ago, I heard about a study of how men view women's bodies. Only six percent of men picked the fashion model body as being the ideal body. The other ninety-four percent wanted a little more meat on the bone. I agree; I

am one of those men who prefer woman to have a little more meat on their bones.

Many women getting into this diet often notice a big change in their menstrual cycle. Sometimes the blood flow stops completely. What is your opinion on this?
Menstruation is an unnecessary thing to start with. It is part of our universal human disease, a female disease. There shouldn't be menstruation, anyway. Menstruation is not the same as ovulation. Although ovulation is very normal, we are so screwed up that we do not have any clarity in this area.

Do you feel it is easier to eat a raw food diet in today's times than it was when you were growing up?
Well, there is certainly more opportunity today. I don't know if it's any easier, but it doesn't bring as many shocked responses from other people. When I was growing up, a big city might have a health food store, but not a raw food store. There is more opportunity for a raw food diet now. Fresh fruit has become more and more available.

Where do you see the raw food movement heading in the future?
I really don't care. I'm not really that concerned about food. Eating naturally isn't all there is. Eating is an outgrowth of my spirituality. Do understand: ultimately, it is all spiritual. I may not be pure, but I am a vegetarian. I don't eat anything that walks, swims, crawls, wiggles, or flies. Life is a precious thing, whether it appears in the form of a bedbug or a giant whale. Even though life is abundant, you can't kill it; it can only change forms. I am a vegetarian out of a reverence for life more than anything else.

Thank you for this interview. In closing, is there anything else you would like to add before we end it?
The one thing that makes the hygienic diet so important is

that it's the only diet that doesn't require anything to die. The apple doesn't kill the tree; the tree produces the apple. We eat the apple, and the tree goes on. This holds true for your vegetables, as well as your tree fruit.

Personally, I know what I'm going to do, no matter what anybody else does. I'm going to do the best I can to follow a raw food diet. Sometimes my best is not very good, but that is what I want to shoot for. Food itself is the least important aspect of my hygienic efforts. I am much more interested in disease and the cause of disease and the cause of health. I am going to follow a lifestyle regime that brings me the highest level of health that I can achieve. I feel better at my worst than most people feel at their best. I feel good all the time.

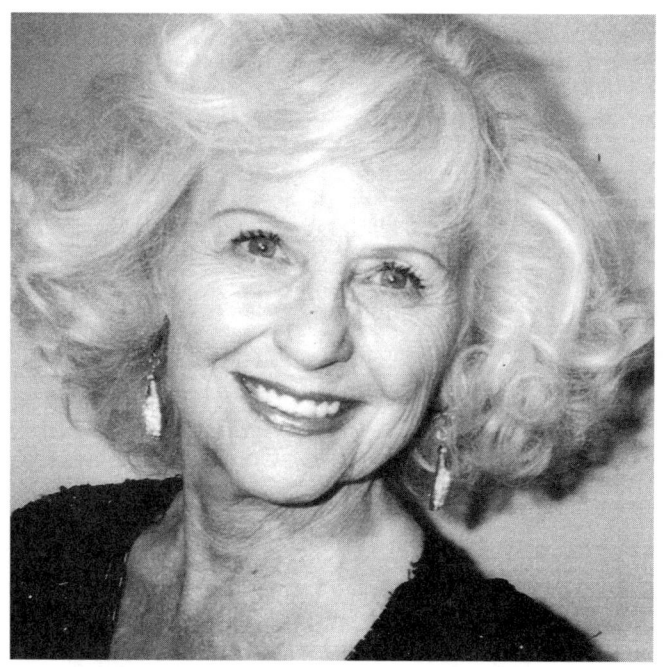

You may contact Virginia at:

Dr. V. Virginia Vetrano
P.O. Box 190
Barksdale, TX 78828

Phone: 830-234-3499
Fax: 830-234-3599
E-mail: vvvetrano@hilconet.com

Or you can visit her health retreat:

Rest of Your Life Health Retreat
P.O. Box 102
Barksdale, TX 78828
Phone: 830-234-3488

Nestled on a crystal clear river in the Texas Hill Country away from the noise, smog and maddening crowds, this retreat provides a peaceful, restful, relaxing and rejuvenating health center.

Drenched in sunshine and warmed by gentle southern breezes, one can simply lie back and enjoy the serenity of Southwest nature in full bloom.

Dr. Vivian Virginia Vetrano

Dr. Vetrano was graduated with honors from Trinity University and then interned at the world famous Dr. Shelton's Health School, studying Natural Hygiene under both Dr. Shelton and Dr. Carl Correlle. They had earmarked her to be the first graduate from the American College of Natural Hygiene, chartered by Mr. C.E. Doolin and Dr. Shelton. She then went on to study chiropractic, receiving the "Keeler Plaque" award upon graduation.

Immediately upon graduation with a D.C. degree, Dr. Vetrano took over as manager and sole Doctor practicing at Dr. Shelton's Health School for the next 18 years, guiding thousands of people through short and long fasts, teaching the principles of Natural Hygiene, editing, writing for and producing Dr. Shelton's *Hygienic Review*, as well as saving lives.

Wanting more knowledge, Dr. Vetrano enrolled in the Kansas City Naturopathic College, and later the United American Medical College in Canada, and further, received a degree in Homeopathic Medicine. Her ability to speak French fluently, quickly opened the door for her to become an international speaker on the subject of Natural Hygiene. She has spoken all over the world many times. In the late 80s and early 90s Dr. Vetrano continued to lecture in the United States and abroad, making several films in California with the late T.C. Fry. She has been specially honored many times.

Dr. Vetrano was President of the American Natural Hygiene Society for two terms and served on its Board of Directors for several years. She was a regular speaker for the ANHS from 1965 until 1987. She was also a certified member of the International Association of Professional Hygienists.

How many years have you been on the raw diet, and what got you into it?
I began eating all uncooked foods in the early 1970s when I quit serving cooked foods at Dr. Shelton's Health School. Actually, I have been eating mostly uncooked foods ever since I became a Hygienist at the age of eighteen.

The first book I read on health was written by Gaylord Hauser. I followed his plan for about six months. Then one day, while I was glancing at the health books for sale in a New York City health food store that I frequented regularly, a man who worked there handed me *Superior Nutrition* by Dr. Herbert M. Shelton and said, "This man's books are the only ones you should be reading." I was startled and happily surprised because the author was from Texas and I was too. So I purchased *Superior Nutrition* by Dr. Shelton and became instantly hooked on Hygiene.

Dr. Shelton's books inspired me because he wrote so honestly and dynamically. When one first studies Dr. Shelton's books, it's like an epiphany - a huge, sudden insight - that at last you are reading the truth. It made sense. He wrote that it is best to live on only uncooked foods, yet he still served very small amounts of steamed vegetables with a large raw vegetable salad at his Health School. The salad was always served first so that the feeders would fill up on raw vegetables before being served small amounts of steamed non-starchy vegetables. Actually, even when I first became a Hygienist, I was already eating only one portion of a steamed green or yellow vegetable a day; I didn't have to break a potato, bread, grain, or legume habit.

One of my prime reasons for eating all uncooked foods was the fact that I did not like to cook. I also knew that cooked foods are less nutritious than raw foods. So why waste time cooking? Additionally, vegetables did not taste good after being cooked, and when I ate cooked foods, my stomach felt warm, heavy, and uncomfortable. When I consumed only uncooked foods, my stomach felt cool, light, and comfortable.

When I decided that it was best for people breaking a fast to eat only uncooked foods, I asked Dr. Shelton to approve my desire to serve all raw foods at the Health School. He wholeheartedly approved it, and after that day, The Health School never served cooked foods on a regular basis. Sometimes, I would feed people a steamed potato or other vegetables on a holiday.

How was your health when you started the diet?
I was in good health when I became a Hygienist, but I was about ten pounds overweight. I was also in good health when I began eating all uncooked foods for good, but I was still too heavy for my satisfaction.

Who are some people who have inspired you to do this?
No one in particular. It came about mainly from studying Dr. Shelton's books and learning about the destruction of nutrients by cooking foods. It was a matter of being educated and making a choice to eat foods which still contain all their nutrients.

I don't think I was so inspired in the sense that I was moved emotionally. There was no one person who motivated me that way. It was a matter of education in the right areas, from diligently studying Dr. Shelton and other Hygienists' books, as well as physiology and nutrition.

You've learned so much over the years. What are a few of the most important things you've learned?
One of the most important things I've learned is that you can never know enough. You must keep learning something new every day. Never quit searching for truth. Besides making life more interesting, it allows you to acquire more facts from which you can reason more accurately. It is very important to realize that every particle of information one picks up makes a difference in the whole. One tiny piece of knowledge here

can add up to an important insight in another area. But you must distinguish truth from fallacy while learning by using your own brain along with the basic Laws of Life. If there is a discrepancy between Natural Law and some new thing being promoted, you have to realize that if the new supposed beneficial "stuff" cannot be used by the body in any way, then it is a poison in relation to the body and therefore harmful and disease-promoting.

Another important thing to learn is that there is no such thing as a "cure." The body is self-healing, and "cures" serve to thwart and interfere with the body's own healing processes.

Another thing that I feel is important when becoming a Hygienist is that you have to learn to stand alone and like it. You cannot expect millions of people out there to coddle you and help you be a better Hygienist. They are eager for you to be proven wrong and just as eager to see you compromise. Perhaps it makes them feel less guilty for what they are doing. Some people are actually uncomfortable eating around you. They want to live without thinking of the future or realizing that their lifestyle is going to hurt them. By your very act of not indulging, you are telling them that they are wrong. No one wants to think that he is wrong. That is why you should never preach Hygiene when you are in the company of non-Hygienists. Learn to keep quiet. That is the best way to keep friends. If they ask you a health question, answer them briefly, and do not elaborate unless they want more. Then recommend a book or tape to them.

One example of how most people react when they first learn about Natural Hygiene or any healthy lifestyle is as follows. My daughter, Dr. Tosca Haag, was home-schooling her children. So she decided to show a group of other mothers who were home-schooling their children the videotape *Diet for a New America* by John Robbins. After viewing this tape and breaking the uncomfortable silence, one of the mothers commented, "Well, carry me out in a body bag." They just did not appreciate the knowledge that the meat diet was harmful to them and to the ecology and cruel and heartless to animals. I guess it was too much of a shock.

Are there any pitfalls that you have learned to watch out for on the raw diet?
The greatest pitfall for most people is in their minds. They do not think about the benefits of the new life; instead, they think mainly about giving up all of their favorite foods and concoctions. In addition, their taste buds are dulled by salt and other condiments. They cannot appreciate unseasoned foods, with the exception of sugary fruits and nuts. I myself had to teach myself to like green vegetable salads. My taste buds enjoyed sweet things such as delicious fresh fruits. I had to make myself eat salads. I copied Dr. Gian Cursio's way of getting children to like salads by permitting myself to eat them with a few dates or raisins. That helped a lot. At the present time, I feed my dog, Peaches, as I would a child. She has a blended salad with two or three dates in it every evening and likes it better that way than she did when I did not put any dates in it.

To conserve nutrients, Hygienists advocate not cutting up salads, unless someone can't chew or must use a blender for some other reason. That makes it more difficult for the neophytes to enjoy vegetable salads. Not only must they forego the dressing, but they also have to cut into a whole tomato, cucumber, celery, and lettuce as they eat. They are just not used to doing that. It's difficult to learn to eat salads without dressings; however, it is best for our health, because salad dressings and sauces complicate the digestive processes and increase the tendency to overeat, both of which can cause fermentation and health problems.

Weight is a big pitfall for many people. Any thoughts about that?

Most people do not know how to eat when they change to all uncooked foods. Eating more than one piece of fruit at a time is inconceivable to them. Therefore, when they begin eating raw foods, they lose weight simply because they do not eat enough fruits and nuts. They can sometimes conceive of having a large salad. While salads are replete with minerals and vitamins, they contain very few calories, so people who consume mostly raw vegetable salads are using more energy in the digestive processes than they are consuming. Naturally, they lose weight. If you are going to eat all uncooked foods, then you must eat a lot of fruit for their caloric and nutritive content. Also, many people are not able to eat sufficiently large portions of fruits or vegetables at one meal. I urge them to eat more than three meals a day.

Most of us are an undisciplined bunch of people who are used to having instant gratification. In order to develop discipline, many people try to limit themselves to only one or two meals a day, but they get in trouble. When you eat only one meal a day, you want to eat everything you like at that one meal. This causes digestive problems for two reasons: (1) overeating, and (2) wrong combinations.

People who are sick when they begin the raw food diet often develop a crisis of elimination. Even latent health problems, such as gastritis or enteritis, will surface. They are frightened, and they often quit the diet since they think that the diet was the cause of their illness. They need the advice of a professional Hygienist, but most of them swear that eating raw food is bad for you.

Naturally, crises and undereating will cause a loss of weight.

Another condition that is latent in many people is mal-absorption. Their digestive powers and absorption are weak, and they will lose weight because of this. Those who persist in eating only the raw foods that they can digest will ultimately begin to gain weight on the same diet on which they lost weight in the beginning.

Dental problems are another big pitfall. Any thoughts?
It's a mistake to think that living on raw foods causes dental problems. On the contrary, it saves your teeth. Teeth begin decaying before we're born because of our mothers' diet. Children's second teeth often come in with cavities. When people are malnourished before birth, they'll have a tendency to have dental caries as they grow older. By the time people begin eating an all uncooked diet, their teeth are already weakened and on the way out; they just did not realize it until the caries surfaced.

The consumption of acid fruits rarely etches the enamel off of teeth. The researchers who published statements to the effect that citrus fruit juices dissolve away enamel did their research using bottled artificial fruit juices with water, sugar, and citric acid. This is just another piece of evidence that you cannot trust modern science, because it performs research using conditions that do not exist in real life, using substances that health-minded people avoid. Ripe oranges, real oranges, and real orange juices are not so acidic as to cause erosion of the enamel. Besides, the body restores the enamel between meals if it has been damaged in any way by normal acid foods. The pH of the saliva ranges from 6.0 to 7.4. For the most part, it is slightly on the alkaline side in a healthy individual.

However, if an individual habitually consumes an **acid-forming** diet in addition to drinking carbonated and acidic juices frequently between meals, the body will not be able to repair the enamel between meals because the mouth is never left empty of the destructors of good teeth - sugars, carbon dioxide, and acids. Those who consume all raw fresh vegetables and fruits normally have saliva that is alkaline. The alkaline medium helps restore the enamel from the abrasive effects of normal chewing.

Saliva actually protects the oral tissues. Saliva washes away pathogenic bacteria and food particles that the bacteria need to eat for survival. Saliva also contains several factors that actually destroy bacteria. These are proteolytic enzymes, thiocyanate ions, and lysozyme. Lysozyme: (1) attacks bacteria, (2) helps thiocyanate ions enter the bacteria, thus killing them, and (3) digests food particles so that the bacteria have nothing on which to feed. They are starved out, metabolically poisoned, and digested. Furthermore, saliva also contains significant amounts of protein antibodies that can destroy oral bacteria, including those that cause dental caries. "Therefore, in the absence of salivation, the oral tissues become ulcerated and otherwise infected, and caries of the teeth become rampant." (*Textbook of Medical Physiology, page 712.*)

Cavities have been known to heal while one is living completely Hygienically. Here is a story that emphasizes the fact that teeth can heal themselves. A man who was a guest at Dr. Shelton's Health School while I was working there showed me a tooth of his that had sealed up its own cavity. The hole was filled in and no longer there. He had not had it filled. He had just left it alone and changed his eating practices and quit drinking Cokes and Pepsis. At that time, it was difficult for me to believe it. But it happened years later to me! When I was around 45, one of my fillings that had been put in when I was in high school fell out. I did not replace it. I kept thinking that I should get it fixed, but there was no pain and I could still use the tooth. It never bothered me, so I just forgot about it. Finally, about fifteen years later when I needed some type of dental work, I asked the dentist to put a filling back in that tooth. He asked me. "What tooth?" I kept pointing to it, but he couldn't see a cavity. Finally, I took the mirror and touched it. He said that the tooth was okay. I was amazed. It had repaired itself!

What are your thoughts about mercury fillings, and what would you replace them with?

It is common knowledge that mercury fillings are toxic and that a small amount of mercury does leak out. My opinion is that a mercury filling is an extra toxic substance that your body has to contend with. If you are healthy, your body may easily eliminate the small amount absorbed each day; yet it is still causing an unnecessary expenditure of energy. Those who are not so healthy may have more symptoms as a result of the mercury. At the same time, just because you have the mercury taken out, that does not mean that all your symptoms will diminish or even go away. I have seen cases where the recovery after the removal of mercury fillings was quick and dramatic, and I have seen cases where there was no improvement whatsoever in health.

I had the mercury taken out of my teeth when I was in school after studying chemistry and before I had read anything about some people's illnesses being attributed to mercury-filled teeth. I just did not want that poisonous substance in my mouth. Gold is not as reactive, and it is perhaps the best choice for most people. But some people have negative thoughts about having metal in their mouths. I have found no composite that does not have some toxic substance in it. I have heard about one made out of coral, but it is not readily available, and even coral has to have something toxic in it to make the coral particles adhere together and harden. Even the light used to harden composites is harmful. I believe that the least toxic way to fill a tooth is with gold, bonded with an *insoluble* resin. If you cannot accept gold or metal in your mouth, then I suggest that you search for the least toxic substance available on the market and request that.

The best thing to do is to live correctly so you won't have to have any more fillings.

There are a lot of controversies in the raw food movement. I will mention some of them, and you can expand a little on each. First of all, what is your opinion

of nuts and seeds?
Nuts and seeds are the best bone builders. The proportion of calcium to phosphorus is the exact proportion that we need for preserving and building bones. The proteins are complete and we do not have to supplement them with anything. They also contain a good supply of the B-Vitamins.

Nuts and seeds are getting a bad name, not because they can't be digested, but because most people have sick digestive organs. People can't digest nuts because their digestive systems have been abused with hot and cold substances, alcohol, cooked foods, tea, coffee, chocolate, chips, other scratchy fried foods, spices, hot peppers, and salt, as well as many other irritants. Consequently, by the time the person arrives at Hygiene's door, they bring a suitcase full of digestive problems. The digestive system is the most abused of all the organ systems of the body. We use it for entertainment, depression, boredom, to get away from it all, and simply for gormandizing. People, in general, habitually overeat. Dr. Herbert Shelton used to say, "We eat but one meal a day - but we take all day to eat it." The mistreatment of our digestive tracts has caused practically everyone in the health movement to think that nuts are indigestible.

Another reason people think nuts and seeds are difficult to digest is that practically no one knows how to eat them properly. Our bodies were expertly designed to digest nuts; people just do not realize it. The glands on the back of the tongue secrete lingual lipase, an enzyme that digests medium and long chain polyunsaturated fatty acids. These are also called the glands of Von Ebner. *There are very few other beings, if any, that have pre-stomach enzymes for the digestion of long chain fatty acids.* Chewing nuts and seeds well saturates them with lingual lipase from the serous glands of Von Ebner. The chewing disrupts the cell walls and mechanically disperses the fat into small droplets upon which lingual lipase acts immediately. Fat (triglyceride) digestion is not inhibited by the acid pH of the stomach. In fact, one can practically state that triglyceride digestion is not inhibited in the stomach at all because of the wide range of pH's in which it can function. Lingual lipase can function in mediums of acidity from a pH of 2 to a pH of 6. Therefore, the activity of lingual lipase continues its enzymic digestion in the stomach. Because of the continued digestion in the stomach, the long chain fatty acids are partly emulsified and digested right in the stomach. If you chew them well, all alone, not using them as a spread on other foods or blended in sauces or with vegetables or fruits, just chewing the nuts or seeds all by themselves, you will often find that you can digest them well. If you grind your nuts, they should still be chewed until they become almost like water before swallowing. Masticating nuts and seeds well improves their digestion, because some digestion will take place in the mouth before it even reaches the stomach, and then it will be continued in the stomach. Also, the saliva that contains lingual lipase continues being secreted for a while after you've finished eating them, and this adds enzymes to the stomach.

Lingual lipase is important because it digests all three types of triglycerides, short, medium and long chain fatty acids. Additionally, gastric esterase (another enzyme) secreted in the stomach digests medium and short chain fatty acids. The digestive enzymes for all types of plant and milk fats are abundant in the mouth, stomach, and duodenum.

The methods of many biochemical reactions are almost like a chain reaction of an atomic mass. Once it gets started, it follows a straight course until the reaction of the atoms is so great that it explodes. The body does not explode, but one trigger leads to another just as regularly as the sun rises. For instance, the digestion of triglycerides in the small intestine is facilitated by *hormones* and *sodium bicarbonate* released by the pancreas. But for this to happen, the following things must be occurring. Digestion must already be in progress as follows: (1) The pH of the stomach must be acidic, (2) digestion must have proceeded until there are essential amino acids from the breakdown of proteins (nuts and seeds are abundant in essential amino acids), and (3) there must be fatty acids and monoglycerides in the gastric juice chyme that reaches the duodenum. Nuts and seeds, because of their high protein content as well as high fat content, are good triggers which cause the small intestine to prepare for their digestion even before they are emptied from the stomach. With those three conditions in place, the mucosa of the duodenum releases cholecystokinin and secretin, which are hormones that are essential for the digestion and absorption of fats. When released, these two hormones work as if they had brains in each atom of secretion.

This is very important information, because knowing that all these reactions are taking place to digest good, raw fats and proteins will help you understand that nuts and seeds can be easily digested. The body is designed anatomically and physiologically with the structures, enzymes, and hormones to do so. Our anatomic and physiological attributes are extremely proficient in the work of digestion and absorption, and the body digests nuts and seeds in less time than anyone could imagine. It has been demonstrated in the laboratory how quickly it does so.

To give you an idea of how the body coordinates its digestive activities, I will describe the two hormone triggers that cause reactions to happen. The first is **cholecystokinin**, and the second one is **secretin**.

Cholecystokinin causes:

(1) the release of enzymes from the exocrine portion of the pancreas (not from the Isles of Langerhans, which secrete insulin);

(2) the release of a large number of electrolytes, the main one being sodium bicarbonate. This is necessary to alkalinize the acid contents being pumped into the duodenum from the stomach. Digestion in the small intestine takes place in an al-

kaline medium;

(3) sustained gallbladder contractions to empty the stored bile into the intestine;

(4) synthesis and release of bile, phospholipids, and cholesterol from the liver. These are all needed for the emulsification and absorption of fats.

One difference between **secretin** and **cholecystokinin** is that secretin is only released by the duodenum when new acid chyme enters the proximal duodenum (close to the exit of the stomach), whereas cholecystokinin is released when food is still in the stomach. In some instances, they cause the same actions to take place.

Secretin:
(1) helps ensure the alkalinity of the small intestine so that intestinal digestion can proceed normally;

(2) is specific for the release of pancreatic electrolytes (atoms or molecules with an electric charge).

Like all other foods, triglycerides must be broken down into smaller particles in order to be absorbed. Triglycerides are enzymatically broken down into fatty acids and glycerol. This process is called hydrolysis because water is added to lyse or split larger molecules. They must then be rendered soluble. Tri- and di-glycerides are not soluble; therefore, they cannot be absorbed. Although tri- and di-glycerides cannot pass through the intestinal wall, monoglycerides can, on one condition - the glyceride must be attached to the middle carbon of the glycerol portion. The glycerol carbon chain contains three carbon atoms, so the monoglyceride must be attached to the middle one. You can think of a monoglyceride as "T". The top of the "T" is the glycerol portion, with one carbon on the end of each side of the cross bar and one in the middle. The stem or the trunk of the T tree is the monoglyceride attached to the middle carbon. Therefore, in this position it can be absorbed. If the fatty acid were attached to the number 1 or number 3 carbon, it would not be absorbed.

Another way that a fatty acid can be absorbed is by becoming protonated by acquiring an additional positively charged proton. If it is combined with a proton or hydrogen atom, it can pass through the mucous membrane by diffusion as free monomers.

The following quotation from a reliable source demonstrates that long chain fatty acids attached to the middle carbon of glycerol and protonated fatty acids can be absorbed very quickly within a short space of time: "It has been shown that 75 *grams* (2.645 ounces) of long chain fatty acids can be absorbed from the aqueous phase as monomers of 2-monoglycerides and protonated fatty acids within four hours by 120 centimeters (3.908 feet) of small bowel." (26) The author writing about the experiment remarked: "This is a formidable accomplishment, considering the fact that the maximum concentration of oleic acid in water is 80 micro-molar and the solubility of glycero 2-monooleate is only 5 micro-molar." (32)

We can understand now that medium and long chain triglycerides are partly hydrolyzed in the mouth, throat, and stomach. Some short chain fatty acids are even absorbed from the stomach. Fat digestion continues in the small intestine by pancreatic lipase and intestinal esterase.

The following is another important quotation regarding the pH changes in the intestinal tract: "pH Changes: Sodium bicarbonate released by the pancreas increases the duodenal pH to the activity level of pancreatic lipase (pH 5.5 to 6.5). Although this is still below optimal pH for pancreatic lipase, such an excess of lipase is secreted (a 1,000 fold excess) that *under optimal conditions, 100 kg of tryglycerides could be hydrolyzed in 24 hours instead of the ingested 100 grams of fat in a normal diet."* [Italics are Dr. Vetrano's.]   100 kilograms = 220 pounds!

I just wanted to impress upon you that we all have the apparatus for digesting the fat and proteins of nuts and seeds; the apparatus is just out of order.

Do not be concerned about the enzyme inhibitors. Trypsin inhibitor in nuts and seeds can be digested in the stomach by the enzyme pepsin, a very potent enzyme. Trypsin is secreted in the *small intestine*, and the trypsin inhibitor in nuts is denatured and its activity destroyed before it has a chance to inactivate our own pancreatic trypsin by the time the nuts reach the small intestine. *Besides, there is no evidence in humans that plant trypsin inhibitor inhibits human trypsin.* The experiments were conducted on rats. There are enzymes in foods themselves that partially digest the enzyme inhibitors before we eat them, and this continues in the stomach before the acid juice denatures them.

What is your opinion of grains and legumes?
We all know that people can live on them, but the question is, can people actually be superbly healthy by partaking of grains, especially a lot of them? The answer is no. A diet of pure grains is acid-forming, and it does not supply the proper proportion of the alkaline minerals to balance the acidic ones. They are low in calcium and iron and very high in phosphorous. In addition, being already low in calcium, grains contain phytic acid. Phytic acid robs you of what little calcium the grain you eat contains by combining with it in the gut and rendering it un-absorbable. Phytic acid also combines with the calcium from other foods in the intestines, rendering the calcium from these other foods un-absorbable.

There are some scientists who believe in the atomic transmutation of some elements in the living body. It has been shown that magnesium can be changed into calcium within the cells of chickens. If this is true for the human species, then this negates the effect of phytic acid because there is a lot of magnesium in grains. On the other hand, as Dr. Shelton wrote, orphans fed only oatmeal in England all developed rickets. However, other things such as sunshine, outdoor exercise, and even milk were also missing. Either humans cannot internally transmute elements, or perhaps babies and children have not yet matured enough to do so. Supporting the immaturity idea is the fact that the myelination of nerves is not complete until the age seventeen or eighteen, and the pancreases of babies and children do not secrete adequate pancreatic amylase to digest the great quantities of starches fed to them until they are around three or four years old.

If you eat grains at all, you should only eat them one time per day, combined with a huge raw vegetable salad. You will be better nourished by combining them with raw vegetable salads but, nevertheless, the cooking itself changes nutrients into toxins. Although you are better off than a meat eater, the cooking destroys essential fatty acids and other nutrients and turns fats into poisons. Do you want that?

Back in the late 1960s, a famous woman claimed that whole wheat was the perfect food, and she was going to prove it by eating only whole wheat while walking from New York to California. Dr. Shelton advised her that she could not do it, but said that if she wanted to use whole wheat, she should at least eat a large quantity of raw vegetables with the wheat. "No," she said, "I want to show people that whole wheat is a perfect food in itself." She refused to eat salads. She collapsed before she even got to Chicago.

Aside from the fact that we are neither herbivores nor grain eaters by nature, there are many other reasons why we should not eat grains or legumes such as beans, peas, and lentils. Grains and legumes are not easily digested by the human organism. When it comes to nuts and seeds, we have all kinds of machinery in place for their digestion at each part in the digestive tract, but grains and legumes cannot be accommodated very well, and they also contain anti-nutrients.

The following reasons are good enough for me to refrain from eating them:

(1) The human species does not have the enzymic capacity that the cow or other herbivorous animals do. Humans secrete only enough salivary amylase to handle the small amounts of starches and sucrose in our natural foods, as in fruits, and nuts and seeds, which contain about 20% carbohydrate, most of it in the form of sugars, and only a small amount in the form of starch. Nuts and seeds are easier to digest than starches, provided that the individual has not ruined his or her digestion by abuse of the organs of digestion. Only a small amount of salivary amylase is needed to digest the remaining starch of nuts and seeds.

(2) All starches including potatoes are composed of two types of starch: a) **amylose**, and b) **amylopectin**.

If you have studied food combining a little bit, you realize that there is a specific enzyme to commence the digestion of a specific food, and even specific enzymes to continue the digestion of a particular food and to break specific bonds until the food is small enough and in a state that can be absorbed. Amylose is digested by salivary amylase and pancreatic amylase. Yet the amount of amylose in starches is only 25%, whereas the amylopectin content is about 75% and its molecular weight is extremely high, ranging from 10 to the 5th, 6th, 7th, and 8th power. Cereals are practically indigestible because they contain amylopectin only. They are called the "waxy" cereal starches.

The simple sugars in amylose are bonded (linked) to each other with a special type of glucosidic bond (type alpha 1- 4). The alpha 1- 4 bond can be digested only with the enzyme **amylase**. On the other hand, **amylopectin** has a different type of link or bond that cannot be digested by amylase. About every 25th glucosidic bond requires a specific enzyme to break, separate, or digest the alpha 1- 6 type of connection. Amylase digests polysaccharides down to maltose, maltotriose, and can digest small branched tri-, tetra- and penta-polysaccharides that contain small amounts of glucose.

If combined correctly and eaten very sparingly, the 25%, amylose portion of the starchy food can be digested by alpha amylase secreted in the mouth and pancreas. However, the specific, different alpha 1- 6 linkages of amylopectin are not affected by alpha-amylase, so they cannot be digested until they reach the jejunum where the **enzyme isomaltase** that can split the alpha 1- 6 bonds is secreted. Meanwhile, bacterial decomposition of the **amylopectin** portion, which comprises 75% of all starches and 100% of cereals, is very likely to occur in the stomach and upper small intestine. The fermentation products of bacterial activity in the intestinal tract are highly toxic alcohols and acids. Overeating or even moderately eating starches tends to enervate and intoxicate and lead to arthritis and other even more serious diseases.

Did you ever wonder why so many people have trouble with pulses such as peas, beans, lentils? It is because the digestive remnants of pulses, after alpha-amylase has partially digested them, are oligosaccharides (a polysaccharide with only a small number of sugar units in the carbon chain) containing two to ten glucose residues of the raffinose family; raffinose itself, stachyose, and verbascose. *These oligosaccharides are small polysaccharides containing alpha-galactoside links (connecting sites or bonding sites) that cannot be digested by the human intestines because humans have no enzyme to disconnect the bonding sites.* If we can't do it, the bacteria are happy to do it. Therefore, many people suffer with gas after eating them simply because we were not designed to eat them.

Starches such as grains, legumes, and some roots are called complex carbohydrates because they really are very complex. We were not designed to eat them. Fruits contain simple sugars that are easily digested by the human digestive system. If very small amounts of grains are eaten, digestion of these may be completed in the small intestine by isomaltase which is designed to digest the alpha 1-6 glucose stub, and the oligosaccharides (small numbers of sugar molecules) are digested by maltases (aka as glucosidases) of which there are three. But you must realize that you will have to accept the consequences of eating foods that decompose easily before they arrive at the small intestine where the enzymes that finish their digestion are located. However, the peas, beans and lentils contain substances that are not digestible.

Newborn babies cannot digest starches at all because the amount of alpha amylase produced by the pancreas is too small for starch digestion. Nutritional studies of newborns noted that there is no glucose in the blood after babies are fed starch. It will ferment in the baby's intestinal tract causing, colic, pain, gas, sleeplessness, and crying. The fermentation products are very toxic to babies and cause serious diseases that could be avoided by using fruits instead of starches. Other evidence of immaturity in newborns is that their brains are not completely developed, and many neurons do not have myelin sheaths to protect them yet. I even think that the blood-brain barrier is not mature enough in babies and young children to discriminate between substances needed in the brain and those that it does not want.

Babies should not be fed starches before the age of three to four years old. Never is even better. The pancreas does not produce alpha-amylase in large enough quantities until the age of three or four. The best carbohydrates to feed babies are sweet fruits.

What is your opinion of an all fruit diet?
I definitely advocate fruitarianism. It is the diet to which we are specifically adapted. It is the most pure and most non-toxic diet on which one could live. It is the only diet that helps to pro-

mote superlative health. However, many people do not understand what it takes to be really healthy. No diet *alone*, however perfectly designed for us, can produce superlative health. You need all the other requisites of health, such as sunshine, rest, sleep, exercise, emotional poise (equanimity), comfortable temperature, pure water, freedom from poisonous habits, cleanliness of body and home, financial and personal security, and loving family and friends.

There are great numbers of people out there promoting the raw diet as the only thing needed to become supremely healthy. They fail to tell people that they need to give up coffee, cigarettes, alcohol and other poison habits and to supply all the other needs of a healthy life. Some raw fooders themselves think that to become a super healthy person, all you have to do is eat all raw. Those raw fooders who continue using over-the-counter and prescription drugs and a host of other enervating things and influences will be sorely disappointed when they discover that they are still sick. The same goes for all those who think that they can burn the candle at both ends - raw fooders, Hygienists, and other health-minded people alike. They never sleep or rest enough, yet they wonder why they are tired all the time. "I'm eating right!" they exclaim, as if that is supposed to make them super-people by itself.

What is your opinion of sprouts?
I do not advocate sprouts. Young plants secrete large quantities of toxins to ward off insects and other plant predators. These toxins are irritants and stimulate those who consume them. The organism can't use those toxins and has to cast them out at the expense of the consumer. Therefore, nerve energy is lost and these types of products promote toxemia.

You can taste the disagreeable pungent, tangy, and bitter quality when you eat them. That alone should give you a warning sign. Your own taste buds, if unperverted, will tell you what food is fit for you and what isn't. Listen to your own body signals. Most sprouts do not taste good, and I could not sit down and make an entire meal of them if I tried, even if I added a dressing or dates to mask the flavor. In contrast, I can easily make an entire meal of one type of fruit and feel like I had banqueted on the most delicious epicurean meal in the world.

The toxic matter in sprouts varies and differs at different stages of growth. When plants feel endangered, the toxins are increased to prevent insects and animals from eating them before they have had a chance to reproduce. For instance, if you pick off only one or two leaves of lettuce, rather than taking the entire plant, the next time you return for more leaves, they will all be too bitter to eat. Plucking the leaves alerts the plant - it feels threatened and endangered. It secretes poison into each leaf to protect itself. There is a tree in Africa which giraffes frequently feed upon, and it only tolerates the giraffe eating it for about thirty minutes. If the giraffe does not quit eating on that tree before thirty minutes, one more bite is toxic enough to make it very sick or even kill it.

I have always contended that sprouts are toxic, and if you want them, no more than a small amount or garnish should be eaten. Many people have been sickened by eating or drinking juices made from sprouts. If you continue drinking juices containing an abundance of sprouts for long, you are in danger of developing arthritis or any other serious condition to which you have an inborn tendency.

The toxins in sprouts, as I said before, create an emergency in the body. It senses the unfitness of the poisonous substances all over the system. The entire system has to go to work to get rid of them. It's like having to put out a fire. These toxins cause urgent physiological activity that waste our nerve energy and damage cells. The individual who eats the sprouts becomes hyper and has a false sense of being energetic and really healthy, but this is the same as getting a caffeine kick or the kick of salt or getting "high" from any other stimulant. The differences between one stimulant and another vary according to how much you eat or drink and how toxic the substance is. Therefore, sprouting is not the answer when it comes to grains and legumes.

Everyone knows that when people are suddenly deprived of their habitual dose of alcohol, coffee, or cigarettes, they go into a great mental, physical, and physiological depression called withdrawal. If sprouts are suddenly withdrawn from people who eat large salad bowls full of them, they, too, will experience withdrawal symptoms. They often do not recognize them as withdrawal symptoms; they just feel that they are having a bad day and attribute it to something else because the symptoms might be mild. They will feel let down, especially those who use sprouts to the exclusion of lettuce or other vegetables in the diet.

I disagree with those people who say that if you eat grains and legumes at all, you should at least eat them sprouted. We were not meant to eat grains, legumes, or sprouts at all. We are neither grain nor grass eaters by nature; we do not have the anatomy or physiology for it. Therefore, sprouting is not the answer when it comes to grains and legumes. Just leave them alone. They were not meant for humankind.

What is your opinion of Natural Hygiene?
I have strived to live completely Hygienically since the age of eighteen. I will be 74 in November, 2002. I have found no error in *pure* Natural Hygiene as taught by Dr. Herbert M. Shelton, only in those who misuse and misinterpret it. Natural Hygiene as taught by those in the now-defunct Natural Hygiene Society is not genuine Hygiene. It is a mug-wump, compromised version. Hygiene was once again sabotaged.

To be a Hygienist, you have to be "in this world, but not of this world," and not many people are capable of doing that. It is a difficult road to travel even for the professional. Many people fail to understand Hygiene because of the untruths pounded into their heads about health and disease from kindergarten through college. Then when they do search for health, there are so many books out there on health that people become confused. They can't tell what is genuine truth and what is not. A lifestyle that is not based on human physiology and its needs cannot be "the truth." If you will notice carefully, most books on health today are written with the goal of selling something artificial, not merely a lifestyle.

A person searching for the road to genuine health should become serious and *study*, not just read, the principles of Natural Hygiene. Natural Hygiene was based on the needs of the body from the beginning. If you do not understand the principles of Hygiene, you cannot possibly carry out the lifestyle properly. It is a way of life, a life-style. It is an entire program which is much more than just a raw diet. If health seekers go on the raw diet only and get sick anyway, they blame the diet, when that probably played a minor role in their development of disease. If you want to be healthy, you have to live healthfully in all ways.

Let me reiterate: most people do not understand Hygiene because they have only heard about it and have never really given it a chance by studying it or living it correctly. Natural Hygiene is a complete way of life based on the Laws of Nature, and not just eating a raw diet. Those who denigrate Natural Hygiene have misconceptions about it. But it is a life in harmony with our physiological needs. Most other "health" books include some Natural Hygiene but with adjuncts, herbs, and some type of therapies to go with it. Well, that's not Hygiene. Hygienists do not sell "cures," and Hygienists think that anyone who tries to "cure" a disease is still thinking with the erroneous ideas of the Middle Ages or even earlier. Only ill-taught and irrational minds try to "cure" disease.

The body heals itself when you remove the causes of disease and supply the conditions of health. It is as simple as growing a plant or making a plane fly. Give the plant what it needs, and it grows and reproduces. Given the right conditions and a good pilot, the plane will fly. Similarly, given the right conditions, healing is a spontaneous biological process that continues until health is reestablished. Just as an airplane can be hijacked and purposely brought down, killing thousands of people, the body can be easily sabotaged with "healing agents" that prevent the very processes the body instituted to re-establish health. Every so-called "cure" is actually a deathblow to millions of body cells, just as an airplane exploding in a big building is a deathblow to the building and many people inside it. The Health Seeker thinks that he or she is closer to health with "cures," but in reality, the Health Seeker is getting closer to death, precisely because of the "cure." All cures waste nerve energy and promote enervation and toxemia.

I want to emphasize that if Natural Hygiene were understood and correctly practiced by all the nations, the whole world could be brought back to its pristine health and happiness in a shorter time than it took for us to degenerate into the physical and mental cripples we are today.

What is your opinion of supplements?

Supplements are never needed. I do not believe that any supplement has anything to offer in helping people keep healthy. On the contrary, I truly believe they are all toxic. No matter how you look at it, no matter how they are prepared, they are still not natural foods. The particular substances in them that are supposed to do so much for you are artificial chemicals or fragments of real foods. Not only are they toxic, but they also upset the balance of Nature. Vitamins are used in proportion to one another and in proportion to the minerals in the diet. If you eat one, you create a demand for another and can actually cause a deficiency because of this.

People want to feel "protected" against disease, so they purchase supplements galore. They have the idea that every disease is a deficiency disease, yet they do not want to stop eating denatured foods or doing things that are making them sick. Supplements make people feel as if they are nourishing their bodies. But they are not; they are malnourishing themselves. The manufacturers of supplements have exaggerated the depletion of our soils and convinced everyone that our foods no longer contain sufficient vitamins and minerals. Even though our foods may contain fewer nutrients than they used to, they still contain adequate nutrients for superior health. People forget that Nature is lavish; there is always more than we actually need. We destroy the nutrients in our foods by exposing them to oxygen, heat, and light.

Nature provides an abundance of all nutrients in all foods. When Nature produces something, it is profuse. For example, billions of sperm are wasted to make just one baby. Thousands of pecans are produced by one tree, when it takes only one to make a tree. Likewise, there are many more minerals and vitamins in our foods than we actually need every day. *The main reason there is no value in our foods today is the destruction of nutrients caused by cooking.*

Cutting, blending, chopping, drying, and mincing also destroy the food value. Raw food gourmet chefs make beautiful salads, pies, pizzas, drinks, and everything else without cooking, yet even though they are tasty and "sooooo delicious," much of the food value has become oxidized and destroyed in their storage and preparation before you get to eat it.

There is plenty of nourishment in the foods we purchase if we eat them as they are, without changing their texture or structure in any way, except by biting or cutting into them and eating them bite by bite. If you must blend your food because of stomach or teeth problems, then make only enough for one meal at a time. It is best not to store leftovers. If you do store foods, keep the time you store them down to a minimum; no more than an hour or two. Use containers that fit the amount of juice or food to be stored. Fill the container to the brim, then cap it to prevent any more oxygen from getting to the food, and refrigerate it.

Even though there may be fewer minerals and vitamins in today's foods, there are still enough to sustain us and help produce worldwide superior health if we quit destroying them in the kitchen. By all means, eat organically grown foods when you can get them.

What is your opinion of eating seasonally?
It is not necessary to eat seasonally, but I think it is good, because many foods will be locally grown and therefore probably won't be contaminated with as many chemicals that preserve them for shipping. But if you can get organically grown foods, particularly fruits, that have been ripened to their maximal extent possible before shipping from any place on this earth, then I see no reason why we should not partake of them. In the beginning, the earth had a spring-like temperature. All foods were attainable all year round. Therefore, we should not become attached to seasonally produced foods from a physiological basis. We were built to eat all kinds of fruits and to have them all the time.

Some animals in the wild, particularly the apes, are starving because they are grazers. Normally, when one crop of a certain fruit is harvested by their act of eating it, they move to another location for another type of fruit that is ripening. But when agribusiness took over the land, their trees were plowed up. They have nowhere to go to eat fruits that ripen at different times. We are in a similar situation. No longer does everything grow where we live all the time. If we want to eat the foods to which we are adapted, then we have to accept foods that are grown elsewhere or eat only frozen crops, which I do not think is ideal. I grant you that imported fruits are not as ripe and plentiful in sugars and vitamins as they could be if they were allowed to stay on the tree longer. Some of the fruits will be more acidic, but if we let them ripen well before refrigerating, they will still furnish us with all the nutrients we need to promote health.

I think we should try to avoid products that have come from South America, because we don't know what type of insecticides, herbicides, or other methods have been used to preserve them. When I purchase strawberries or other foods, that sit in the refrigerator for weeks without rotting, particularly fruits, "I smell something rotten in the air," and I don't want to have anything to do with them. Strawberries used to go bad within a week - but when they last for a month, something is definitely abnormal.

What is your opinion of fasting?
Genuine fasting is so beneficial in the care of the sick that were more people to understand it, they would never say fasting is "dangerous." Fasting (water only) is not usually dangerous, but it could be if you don't have proper supervision. You can never get the same good results by going on a juice diet, which is often wrongly called a "juice fast." If you are drinking juices, you are eating. That is not fasting. Going on juice diets is better than doing nothing, but the recovery of severe chronically ill patients by drinking juices is so slow and health is not as forthcoming as it could be by the intelligent use of a genuine fast. As a result, they give up and return to their wrong living habits and, worse, to medications. Another serious consequence of juice dieting is that some people carry it out too long and suffer from a protein deficiency. They continue being active without securing the rest and sleep they need to get well. When their symptoms persist, they think they need detoxifying again, and again start only juices. Thus, they keep this up for years, seriously depleting all their reserves until they are walking skeletons and can't fast. Juicing is not the road to health, and detoxifying can be carried to harmful extremes.

Those who have a thorough knowledge of *genuine* Natural Hygiene to begin with, then a thorough knowledge of pathology, physiology, and pharmacology, are the proper ones to conduct fasts. This does not mean that everyone will get well, because the pathological and structural changes in many people are too severe to reverse. But even in some cases where I thought reversal was impossible, the impossible happened - they got well! Miracles do happen.

Many individuals fast on their own after reading only one or two books, without ever having studied fasting in-depth or ever having fasted under supervision. Not being trained in physiology or pathology, they are unable to correlate the changes happening with the fasting state, nor are they able to determine if it's a disease symptom or a serious disease process. They do not know how to conduct their own fast, yet they sometimes try to conduct another person's fast. They do not understand the importance of resting while fasting. They drink too much water, take enemas, exercise, and often continue working. Some stay in the sun too long. There are some neurological conditions that are hurt by staying the hot sun too long, and in general, no one should even sunbathe when it's extremely hot, whether fasting or feeding. This is especially true while fasting. Because people when fasting only sleep part of the night, they tend to keep the light on and read. They watch TV all day, or read and sit up and talk all day long. The results achieved by the people who do not properly carry out the fast will, of course, be minimal.

All types of rest are necessary while fasting. This means that you must rest physically, mentally, emotionally, physiologically, and sensorially. One is sick because of chronic enervation and toxemia. The only way to regain the function of the enervated system is to rest completely. The toxins will be excreted in proportion to the amount of normal nerve function and organ power at the present time. Resting permits the body to use all of its forces in cleansing, repairing, regenerating, and renewing. *But you have to do it correctly.*

Reading one or two books on fasting does not make you capable of conducting your own fast, particularly if you are sick.

Sometimes, those who are really healthy can fast on their own. They rarely get in trouble. But even those who think they are healthy sometimes develop an unsuspected crisis while fasting which they cannot handle. Three things then take place: (1) They do not know what is going on, and they get confused. (2) Their family and friends frighten them. (3) They become frightened and go to the hospital where they become more frightened and agree to medication and other more harmful treatments. Physicians freak out at the level of ketones and other findings and often prescribe drugs that have nothing to do with the condition of the individual and cause even more problems for the person already in crisis. Disasters may result due to ignorance and fasting without the guidance of someone who is knowledgeable in the process.

Fasting sometimes brings a chronic disease out into the open. An underlying chronic disease is returned to the acute stage. It often surfaces as a crisis, and it indicates that the body is trying to heal it. Those who do not know a serious pathological condition from a crisis often get in trouble due to their lack of knowledge and do the wrong thing. This gives fasting a bad name. But the problem was not caused by the fast; it happened because the person fasting did not have sufficient knowledge to fast alone.

What is your opinion of food combining on a raw diet, and is it necessary?
Yes. If you intend to eat several types of foods together, I think food combining is necessary. Although it is less difficult to combine wrongly when eating all uncooked foods, I still think it's necessary to combine foods properly. For instance, were you to eat a four or five ounce portion of nuts with a lot of dates or other dried fruit, you probably would have discomfort, gas, or both. Bananas and other sweet fruits do not go well with nuts. Even eating avocados with bananas, grapes, and other very sweet fruits causes trouble in many people.

Avocado, being a high fat food, tends to take longer to empty from the stomach. When fruit is eaten with avocado and held up in the stomach too long, it ferments. Green vegetable salads tend to negate the delay of stomach emptying. Therefore, if you eat avocado and greens plus a few pieces of even a sweet juicy type fruit, digestion will be more rapid than if you ate only fruit and avocado.

What is your opinion of physical exercise?
Exercise is not only good, it is very important. Exercise causes every organ and organ system in the body to improve its condition and become stronger. The blood vessels become stronger and more elastic, the bones become larger and stronger, the brain improves and sets up new nerve pathways. Children's minds improve in their development. The heart, lungs, kidneys, gastrointestinal tract, and muscles all become stronger, larger and capable of doing their special jobs of supporting themselves and other organs better. There is not one cell in the body that is not better nourished and improved with judicious exercise. While we are exercising, white blood cells which hide in muscle tissues leave these sites and begin to circulate to help remove toxic debris. Our entire immune system is benefited by exercise. Exercise is good for the elderly as well as the young. Were more people to exercise and get sunshine, there would be less osteoporosis in both genders.

More importantly, exercise is good because it can correct physical deformities when used intelligently. Some babies are born with inverted or everted feet. They can't learn to walk because their feet are turned inward (medially) or outward (laterally). Instead of using braces, which further weaken the musculature of the feet and calves, the proper passive and active exercises can correct the problem. The correct exercise program can correct inguinal and umbilical hernias, fallen organs, and various spinal deformities such as kyphosis, lordosis, scoliosis, and combinations of these. All of this can be done without surgery and its accompanying risks.

Let us not forget the benefits of exercise for beauty. Not all of us are born with perfect physical bodies, but with exercise, small calves can be developed into eye-catching, beautifully proportioned structures that give you greater strength to walk, run, and jump. The thighs and every muscle in the body can be developed to their greatest potential with resistance exercises. The development makes us not only fit but also more beautiful and functionally superior.

Weight training should be done carefully and gradually with correct posture and form. You should seek a good instructor who is an expert in the field. With a good instructor and the correct posture and form, you will not strain any body part. It's fun and invigorating to feel your muscles perform for you as you powerfully will them to.

I do not approve of programs that are intended to build muscle quickly for contests, because they put emotional and physical stress on most individuals. The overwhelming desire to win often causes over training, which sometimes results in serious injuries. Competition puts a mental, emotional, and physical strain on the best of us. We should exercise without taking steroids or supplements. Each person is unique and will make a natural gain in musculature and health within his or her own inherent ability and capacity. So you should exercise, be patient, and enjoy the rewards of health, fitness, and beauty by doing resistance exercises.

What is your opinion of wild foods?
Wild foods are fine, but the ones we have in this area of Texas are neither very appetizing nor palatable, with the exception of pecans and mulberries. The natural cactus fruits have too many seeds and very little pulp, even less than the pomegranate. The cactus plant itself would give us water and vitamins and would be okay if we had nothing better to eat. People usually cook it. So many years have passed since I tasted a cactus plant, I've for-

gotten how it tastes. They have so many thorns that they really intimidate us. The wild greens here are too high in oxalic acid and other pungent substances. The wild persimmons are very tiny and black. They are not really sweet, but they have a pretty good flavor. Be aware, however, that if you eat too many, you will get a good purging. They would make good laxatives. We have pine nut trees growing wild in some areas here. The pioneers are said to have planted them. They taste pretty good, but there are none where we live. The watercress growing by the natural springs is too pungent. I tried it, and I would eat it only if nothing else were available. We have purple flowered, yellow fruited weeds of the nightshade family that even horses, goats, sheep and cows won't touch. We have one longhorn bull whom we call "Wobbles" because as a young calf he got an overdose of a particular poisonous rye grass. It damaged his nervous system. He has to wobble to walk and is so uncoordinated that he often falls. He gets up with great difficulty. We thought he would succumb at an early age because he was not able to get up. But his body rallied and his muscles developed despite a poor nervous system. He seems to be no more wobbly than he was when he was young. He still manages to get to food and water by swaying back and forth and inching along. We have mushrooms galore, but they are indigestible and pass through the digestive tract unchanged; very little of the nutritive value is usable. I have not seen many of the poisonous types here, but then I have not been looking. Dandelion greens are plentiful, but they are bitter and the leaves are very tough. What is left but rocks?

Let us concede that most of us do not live in our *natural environment*. We will have to be satisfied with foods that are imported from other areas. I do not believe in fiddling with genes, but I think that we can take the best fruit of a tree and foster the seed of that fruit tree to get a better plant which produces a superior fruit. I am not one to believe the myth that there is too much sugar in our fruits.

What are your height and weight? Has your weight changed, or were there other changes your body has gone through? How did you handle it?
I am five feet two inches tall. I weigh 92 pounds. I became a Hygienist in order to lose weight, but I still had a difficult time losing weight; I had too many fat cells. My mom said she brought me up on malted milk after weaning me. I even gained weight on fruit. So I had to learn to eat salads. Ugh!

I do not remember any changes that took place in my body other than a larger chest size as a result of strenuous and persistent physical exercise and white hair and wrinkles as I got older. I was an outdoor girl and had far too many sunburns, and supposedly I should have developed skin cancer by now. I've been in contact with indoor city people who very rarely got out into the sun but have developed melanoma and other types of skin cancer. Their diets were conventional and animal foods predominated. I'm comparing lifestyles and not trying to hurt anyone or brag. And I'm keeping my fingers crossed.

Did you ever really get sick or have a really bad detox?
I never had a bad detox from fasting. In fact, I fasted so often to keep my weight down in my early life, my body would not let me fast anymore; I would never lose my hunger. I know what genuine hunger is because I taught myself to discover it after reading about it in Dr. Shelton's books when I first became a Hygienist. When I tried to fast, I'd get hungry and I would have to eat around the fifth day every time. Sometimes my hunger would never subside, or if it did, it would subside for only one day and then return very strong. I once fasted eleven days with my hunger growing stronger every day. I finally broke that fast. During that fast, I felt hunger not only in my mouth and throat but also throughout the entire body. Dr. Shelton had never heard of that, but I know it occurs. With few exceptions, the body forces you to eat when nutrients are needed, whether you want to or not. You feel like a hungry lion in a cage stalking back and forth.

Your desire to fast is so strong, you put yourself in a mental cage and stalk back and forth in your mental cage until your body forces you to break the cage apart and get food. After the eleven day fast and being hungry every day, I decided that I had fasted too often and too close together, so I did not fast any more to lose weight. About twenty years later, I decided to fast because I was not working any more and I needed a good rest. I did just fine for thirty days. No crises, no hunger, just a good, relatively easy fast. I probably had recuperated the nutrients I needed to fast with and I did not get hungry until around the end.

There is no such thing as a bad "detox." Detoxification takes place throughout the fast whether or not you have a strong elimination crisis. You can get well without ever having a crisis. Crises, or what the layman calls a "bad detox," are actually "good detoxes" if they occur. They usually occur when the body aims all its energy at one particular pathological problem such as when a chronic disease is reversed to the acute stage of the disease. It also happens when the mucus and serous membranes and the salivary glands need to assist the primary organs of elimination such as the liver or kidneys. One of the basic reasons for a crisis of elimination is that the body has no enzymes to biodegrade all the man-made chemicals in this age that somehow get into the body via the mouth, or absorption through the skin and mucous membranes. Since it has no enzymes in the liver or body cells to biodegrade the toxic substance into something that the lungs or kidneys can eliminate, it has to chuck it out via a skin rash, or vomiting, or by secreting mucus throughout the entire intestinal tract and upper respiratory tract, or by other vicarious means. Children almost always vomit gastric juice, and they have a tendency to excrete toxins through their skins. Emotional people are the ones who usually have a salivary crisis. Their glands secrete an enormous amount of bad-tasting saliva, and the individual is compelled to expectorate day and night. When the liver is secreting a lot of toxic bile, it backs up into the stomach and causes vomiting. I repeat, there is no such thing as a bad "detox." However, if they occur at the end of a very long fast, and the individual is very weak, it is best to break the fast.

Crises are always, in all conditions, aimed at returning the body to its pristine cleanliness and health.

Do you eat 100% raw foods, and if so, for how long?
I do not eat cooked foods. I have been on all uncooked foods since around the 1970s.

What is your average daily diet like? What do you eat and how often?
I eat very little, and very little at a time. According to the new definition of a Breatharian, I am almost there. I eat no more than about ten to eleven ounces of food at a meal. The least I eat at a meal is one and a half ounces to two ounces. That is my nut or seed meal. I eat fruits, nuts, and sesame and sunflower seeds, carrot juice or vegetable juice, and once in a while, lettuce. My meals are spaced about three hours apart, depending upon hunger. I fix my dog a blended salad every day and I nibble on it before I put it into her bowl. It consists of lettuce, red bell pepper, raw corn, carrot, celery, and three dates.

What is your favorite food?
Any food when I am hungry. I make myself wait until I am ravenous. Then I start fixing my meal. The foods I like best are melons, bananas, dates, oranges, and fresh figs. I like cherimoyas, but I can rarely get good ones unless I go into San Antonio.

Out of all foods, what do you think is the most important?
I like that question because I can answer it thusly: people keep thinking that one food is more important than all the others, but it is the *total diet* that counts. My main argument, however, is that health is not built from merely eating raw foods. Eating raw foods exclusively does not insure health, although it is a major step in the right direction. The most important issue is

our entire lifestyle. Our entire lifestyle, not just our diet, has a bearing on our health. You could be eating 100% raw but not be getting enough sleep and rest, and you would soon find yourself sick. We need to supply all the needs of physiology, not just one. If we fail to supply one, or supply too much of any of them, we will get sick. We will stay well when we supply all the conditions of health and avoid all poison habits, and that includes emotional and mental poison habits.

How are your health and energy?
I have more stamina than most 74-year-old people, but not as much as I had when I was 65. I have lots of energy when I need it most, however. The following story will demonstrate what I can do.

My dog, Peaches, loves to hunt. She is a mix of a small poodle and Lhasa apso. Sometimes, I let her stay in the yard with a fifteen foot chain dangling loose on her, so I can grab it if she starts to run after some animal. I also keep a loose chain on her so she will get caught in a fence or something before she runs too far away from home. If she gets caught far away from home, it's very difficult to find her, because she likes to hunt in thick brush.

One hot summer morning when I thought she was tied, I went about my work not being concerned that she would go hunting. But suddenly, I noticed that the primary tie chain had no Peaches at the other end. When she had been gone over one hour, I knew that she was caught on something, but where? There is a lot of countryside around here, and she can squeeze through fences. I called her and looked under the house and all around the yard and barn area, but I could not find her.

I picked up my granddaughter's school friend, Alisa, to help me. To save time, she was going to walk through the woods with me, with each of us covering a fifty foot span, back and forth, but it was so hot, I had to keep sending her back for water. It was 109 degrees Fahrenheit, one of the hottest days in Texas last summer. I trudged through the woods and brush for eight and a half hours, not even taking a break to eat. I had to search mostly in the brush because I could easily see around big trees. When the brush got too thick, I had to crawl and sometimes cut my way through in order to determine whether or not Peaches was there.

I could not follow her barks, as I sometimes can, because she only barks when she has an animal treed or when she finds one in its hole, so I had no idea where she could be. She had evidently gotten tangled up on something before she found an animal. I was pretty concerned, because in the past, she has been lanced in her tongue by a porcupine, and she has been doused with skunk perfume. Just recently, she fought a raccoon who was as big as she is. I could hear her yelping; so I ran to the door to let her in, but the raccoon would not let go. When she came in, it came in with her! It was clinging to her like a leech with claws and fangs digging into her. I had to kick him off and then out of the house. What a frightful time I had!

But, back to the search. Peaches is a small dog and not easily found, but I was not going to give up until I found her. With sweat pouring off of me, I kept walking without a break because it was getting late, but I finally had to go home without her. When my granddaughter, Raven, came home from work, I told her that maybe Peaches was under the house and I just couldn't see her. Raven could not see her either, but she got a flashlight and discovered the end of her leash hung up on a nail of the wooden foundation. How we finally had to get her out is another long and harrowing story. From that day on, I call Raven my heroine.

Regarding energy: I walked for over eight hours in the sweltering weather and then worked for two more hours helping Raven as she dug under two big beams before she finally got to the dog. When you get older, you sometimes feel as if you have no energy, mainly because you just don't want to do something, but when stamina is needed, it is there if you've been active and living correctly, in general.

How much sleep do you get, and how much do you think is necessary?
The amount of sleep needed varies for each individual. I think an older person requires more sleep or at least more rest than a younger person does. I sleep about six to seven hours at night and I rest and try to nap twice a day, or more if I'm really tired. If I wake up at night, I usually stay in bed with my eyes closed, resting and thinking positive thoughts.

Although I do not need much sleep, I still require physical rest. If I'm still tired when I awaken, I stay in bed with my eyes closed until I feel completely rested.

Have you noticed any mental changes on the raw diet?
When I was about eleven or twelve years old, I often had a hazy feeling in my head. I never knew what it was until I studied Hygiene. I was consuming a lot of starches and refined sugar, and I believe that I was intoxicated with the various alcohols produced in the gut by bacteria. After I began eating only fresh fruits, non-starchy vegetables, and nuts and seeds, I've never had that drunk feeling again.

When it comes to relationships, many people just beginning a raw diet have problems because their mates do not want to change. Do you have any comments or suggestions?
When I got married, I never had a problem regarding diet. In France, people seem to let one live as he or she wants without interfering. When I ate with my husband, I made a vegetable salad for both of us. We literally had the same meal with the exception of the type of protein. My husband cooked the meat he wanted to eat, and I ate nuts.

I think we should set good examples and try not to push our ideas on others, not even our spouses. When they see how energetic and happy we are and how good we feel, they take notice - especially when they themselves are lethargic and tired most of the time. Sometimes, they will change their own minds and try something different.

Has you attitude towards sex changed over the years?
I found out when I was a newlywed that I had a lot less energy to practice ballet than I did before I got married. I think people would be better off by indulging in sex more moderately.

Do you think it's harder for a woman to eat a raw diet than it is for a man? If so, why?
Under the proper circumstances, it is not more difficult for a woman to eat a raw diet than it is for a male. In fact, it is often more difficult for a male because males sometimes especially feel a loss of strength when they stop consuming meat and cereals. The only reason it's more difficult for a woman is that she usually has to prepare the meals for the entire family who perhaps are not yet eating all raw. She will be tempted to eat or at least taste what she is cooking.

Why do you think there are more raw men than raw women?
I have not thought about it, and I do not know.

What are your thoughts about the female menstruation cycle? Do you think it is natural for a woman not to bleed when she is on a raw diet, or should there be blood? Either way you answer, please explain why.
A woman can cease menstruating for two reasons: (1) she is extremely healthy yet still ovulating; and (2) she is toxic, anemic, and malnourished. In the latter case, she will stop menstruating and also cease to ovulate.

There does not have to be blood when the uterus sloughs off its lining. The uterus is engorged excessively, and this causes it to build a thicker uterine membrane than necessary for a fertilized ovum to nest in. When the uterus is excessively engorged and the nidus for a baby is being built, capillaries must grow into the structure to nourish the extra tissues. Since the epithelium is too thick, the capillaries have to be longer and more abundant to nourish all that extra tissue. When the body sloughs it off, bleeding occurs because the tissues and capillaries are excessive. In a genuinely healthy woman, the membranes will slough without bleeding or with very little bleeding for several reasons: (1) the endometrium will not have become overly thickened; (2) the arterioles feeding the capillaries will contract at the proper time and tightly enough to prevent blood from leaking into the endometrium that is sloughing; (3) the capillaries necessary for a less thick endometrium will be fewer and shorter; and (4) by the time the skin begins to slough off, the capillaries will have shrunk along with the dying endometrium. Only a small amount of extra endometrial fluid will slough off.

I think it will take many generations to regenerate strong physical bodies and to reverse the DNA changes that may be the cause of the bleeding. Physiology has become patho-physiology. It's up to us to reverse it.

When I first got my female dog, she must have been about six months old. When she came into heat, she bled so much that she needed a dog belt and pads. Then I put her on an all uncooked diet, and now I have difficulty determining whether she is in heat or not. Only sometimes, do I note a tiny drop of blood on her bedding. There is usually only a little excess of a clear mucoid secretion.

Any comments about PMS and the raw diet?
PMS occurs for the same reason that other ailments occur: poor lifestyle and lack of exercise, sunshine, and emotional balance.

Any comments about pregnancy and the raw diet?
Women give birth much more easily on an uncooked vegetarian diet than they do when eating meat and other cooked

foods. Additionally, there are fewer complications.

Thank you for this interview. In closing, is there anything else you would like to add?
Yes, but I have said enough already. Actually, I was going refute the erroneous thoughts being circulated about the way that fructose supposedly causes a high triglyceride level and is unnatural and harmful, but what I wrote grew and grew until it ended up becoming a chapter for my new book on vegetarianism. So if you really want to know about that, keep in touch with me.

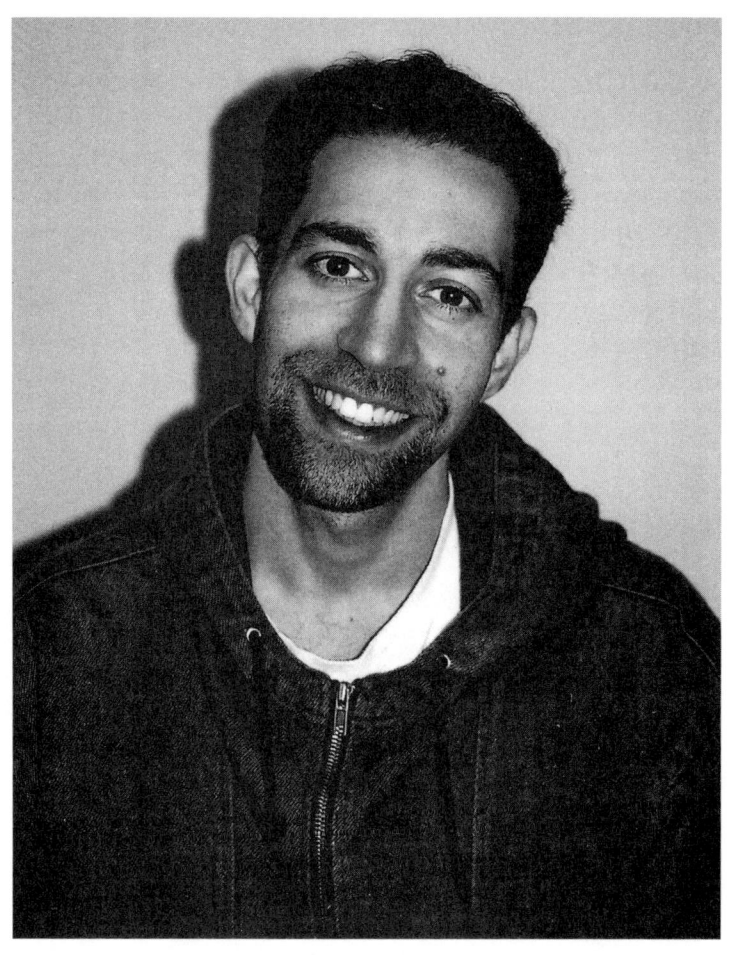

Paul is the author of this book. You may contact him at:

Paul Nison
P.O. Box 443
Brooklyn, NY 11209

Phone: 917-407-2270
Website: www.rawlife.com

Paul Nison

When did you first hear about the raw food diet, and what made you want to try it?
I first heard about the raw food diet around 1993 when I moved to West Palm Beach, Florida. I moved very close to The Hippocrates Health Institute. At the time, I was a vegan. My health had been improving, but it was still not the best. I've always wanted to be the best I can be, so I kept searching. When I found the raw food diet and tried it, it worked for me right away, taking all of my illnesses away.

How was your health before you started the diet?
I was already a vegan, so it wasn't too bad. But I was still suffering from colitis attacks every now and then, however, far less frequently than before having become a vegan. But I wanted never to suffer from a colitis attack or any other disease ever again.

How long did it take you to heal once you started eating a raw food diet?
I was eating mostly raw foods for a good number of years before I went 100%. Until that point, I was feeling better, but not 100% better. Since going 100% raw, I've had some healing (detoxing) episodes, but I would say I was better from day one.

When you tried this diet for the first time, what attracted you to it?
The thought that I would never suffer from disease again was what motivated me to do it.

Who inspired you the most to eat a raw food diet?
I would say my biggest inspiration was not a person, but my illness. I would have tried anything to avoid the pain and to get

better. That was my real inspiration. At the Hippocrates Health Institute, I'd read a few books by Ann Wigmore and Brian Clement. They gave me a lot of needed information, but then I found a book by Joe Alexander titled, *Blatant Raw Foodist Propaganda*. That book listed authors of other books and spoke about the raw food movement. It really inspired me to check out all the information I could find about the raw food diet and lifestyle.

You've learned so much over the years. What are some of the most important things you've learned?
There are so many things. I keep learning; but up to now I would say that making the change to a raw diet has much more to do with the mental than the physical. It's easy to physically pick up a piece of fruit and eat it. But mentally, to deal with people and society when you eat this way, and to keep doing it regardless of what others say about it, is the challenge.

Another important thing people need to understand is that it took a long time to get sick, and you're not going to get better overnight by eating a raw diet. It takes time. So give it time and you will get better. Don't doubt the power of nature. Be positive.

Something I've learned is: this is not about being perfect, it is about being free and happy. Having the correct, complete knowledge will give you true happiness. If you're doing this and are not happy, then you need to learn more about the reasons for doing it. Get the information. Replace the fear with knowledge. If you have any fear, you simply do not have the correct or complete knowledge.

Are there any pitfalls you've learned to watch out for on the raw diet?
Yes; not to think you know it all. No one knows it all. No two people are in the same place at the same time, so there can never be one answer for everyone.

I think each person has to find what works best for him and what doesn't work best. But to stop searching and give up is a pitfall. Hang in there and the answers will come.

I see many people on a raw diet overeating, also eating way too much sweet fruit. From what I see this will only lead to problems and give the raw food diet a bad name.

It's just like the S.A.D (Standard American Diet) where people overeat and eat too much sugar. The only difference is that it's raw. It might not be as harmful as eating cooked food, but just because raw food is high quality doesn't mean we can overdo it and not suffer the consequences. If you do that you will suffer. Your body will tell you the answer to how your doing by how you look.

What is your opinion of nuts and seeds?
They are very helpful to people new to a raw diet. Many people tend to overeat on them. If one gets control over eating them, and gets good quality nuts or seeds, they could be wonderful. Soaking them might really help, especially if overeating them.

What is your opinion of grains?
For some people they can be helpful during the transition. But in the long run, I think anyone would be better off without them. If someone chooses to eat them and feels fine, that's all right. I know many people who are raw and still eat sprouted raw grains and feel fine, but I know many people who don't eat them, including me, and also feel great.

What is your opinion of fruitarianism?
I think greens are very important and I've never met or heard of a long term raw person who ate only fruit and was healthy. I'm not saying they don't exist, but I am saying I haven't heard of them.

What is your opinion of sprouts?
I eat sunflower sprouts mainly for taste. I know the Hippocrates

Health Institute has many studies reporting their excellence for healing. I think they are good, but not needed every single day. I eat them more for taste.

What is your opinion of Natural Hygiene?
I think the Natural Hygiene diet and lifestyle would be great if we were living in nature; but we are not in nature and haven't been living a natural life for a very long time. So, some unnatural things might be needed to help us that Natural Hygiene doesn't agree with. When a person is healthy, I think there is no better way to eat than a natural diet. I've heard people compare Natural Hygiene to living and eating the way the animals in nature do. If that is what is meant by it, I have yet to meet anyone who lives or eats this way.

What is your opinion of supplements?
I don't agree with taking vitamin supplements. I think that's a waste. You can get all the vitamins you need from food. I do believe in super foods. Some people call them supplements, but they are just food in powdered or liquid form.

What is your opinion of eating seasonally?
I think eating this way is the best way to eat if you can do it. It's not too easy in today's world; so do the best you can. That's what I do.

What is your opinion of fasting?
I think the less people eat, the better off they are. Fast as often as possible. Many people can do this physically, but doing it mentally is the hard part because so many people eat for emotional reasons.

What is your opinion of food combining on a 100% raw diet, and is it necessary?
I think food combining is always important and always helpful.

What is your opinion of physical exercise?

I once saw an interview with Jack LaLanne. He said, "Going one day without exercise is like committing suicide." I agree 100%. I think we should all get some form of exercise every day.

What is your opinion of wild foods?
Nutritionally, they are the best. If they taste good and you enjoy eating them, great. The more that people learn to identify wild foods, the better off they'll be in the future.

What are your age, height, and weight?
I'm 5'7" and weigh around 145 pounds. At the time of this interview I'm 31 years young.

Has your weight changed, or were there any other changes your body went through? How did you handle it?
Within the first weeks of going 100% raw, my weight dropped from 140 pounds all the way down to 118 pounds. My energy also dropped, and all I wanted to do was sleep. Getting rest was easy, but dealing with people was the hard part. I decided to avoid people whom I thought would give me a hard time, and when I did have to see them, I made sure I was wearing a lot of clothes. I didn't even want to look at myself in the mirror. But now I wish I had taken many pictures because they would have made some great before and after pictures.

Did you ever get really sick or have a really bad detox during your transition to this diet?
Twice, I had really bad days. They only lasted for one day, twenty-four hours. It was hard, but I made it through. I had the worst headache and was very dizzy and tired. The headache was so bad, I could barely stand. I just kept telling myself, after a good night's sleep, I will be better. I really had to dig deep down inside to muster my will power not to give in and take aspirin. It paid off. Both times, the next morning I felt amazingly well.

Do you eat 100% raw foods, and if so, for how long?
I ate mostly raw food during the first few years, but every night

I would have millet or tempeh. Finally, about five years ago, I went 100% raw and have never looked back. I'm sure, over the years, I've eaten something cooked without realizing it, but I've never eaten cooked food on purpose since going all raw. I've never even had a craving. I think because I took my time and made the change in stages, it wasn't too bad. I see people who do it overnight, but many of them seem often to get cravings for cooked food.

What is your average daily diet like? What do you eat, and how often?
My body is always changing; and because I'm always learning new things, my diet changes as I learn. At present, I'm eating the way I've been eating for the last few years. When I first started, I ate much more. I overate for sure. I also follow food combining concepts much more attentively now. I used to eat raw food prepared from recipes all the time, now I very rarely eat them. Since I travel so often, I don't always eat this way, but I usually eat one or two sweet meals a day and one or two salads a day. I eat about two to four meals a day. I never snack between meals. If I feel hungry, I'll have a green drink between meals. I have a few green drinks a week. I also eat many blended foods. I often blend up my salads. I have gone for months on just blended food. It really gave me the discipline to help me stay focused on my goals.

Is it hard to eat what you want while traveling on the road?
It isn't too bad. There's usually a health food store wherever I go. I can always get a salad. If there is no food for me where I go, I just won't eat. It's no big deal for me. Every now and then something like that happens, and I just fast for the day.

What is your favorite food?
Durian is my favorite, but I really like whatever is in season and is fresh and ripe.

How are your health and energy?
They are good and getting better every day. I hear stories about people who need very little sleep when going raw, but I still like to get a good amount of sleep. I do a lot of work every day and like to get good rest. Much of my work is mental and that takes a lot out of me. I like to think of it this way, for every hour I work, mental or physical, I want to get an hour of sleep. If I work eight or nine hours a day, I'll sleep eight or nine hours. But if I only work a few hours, I only need a few hours sleep. That doesn't happen often because I'm very busy writing books and setting up talks. My health seems to be fine. I do the best I can.

How much sleep do you get, and how much do you think is necessary?
I think it's very easy to under sleep and impossible to oversleep. I do my best to sleep as much as possible and think everyone should. The more we work, the more sleep we should get. The body needs the rest to heal. I would say right now, on average, I sleep about seven to eight hours a night. I can go on much less, but I don't like to unless I really have to. I see under sleeping as a big problem in society. Many healing functions take place during sleep. The blood gets cleaned and the body heals. The amount of time for each person is different. There are no two people in the same place at the same time.

What mental changes have you noticed?
I used to worry a lot. I still worry, but much less and I keep improving. The less I worry, the better I sleep. I can remember things better since going raw, and I can do many things at one time. My mental ability has definitely improved since going raw.

What spirituality changes have you noticed?
Before I was raw, I used to think when we die that's it, that there is nothing else out there. Now, I know there is for sure more out there than we can see. I feel it everyday. The greatest gift I have gotten out of being raw is this newfound love for a higher

power. I know as long as I keep doing things with good intentions, I will get what I deserve. It really helps me love life much more. I say it's a gift, but it is not really a gift. It's natural to think this way, but it's taken away from us when we are born and our bodies are stuffed with cooked food and other junk.

What are your thoughts about relationships? Many people just getting into a raw diet have problems because their mates don't want to change. Do you have any comments or suggestions?
I think the hardest thing is when a couple has kids and one parent goes raw and wants to bring their kids up raw, but the other parent keeps feeding the kids junk. I don't have an answer for this. I guess the best answer right now would be to keep praying; and your prayers will be answered when the time is right. I am lucky. I'm not in this situation, but I see it with many people.

Many people think it would be harder to have a relationship when you eat this way and I thought the same thing, but oh was I wrong. When you eat this way and find a partner who understands and eats this way too, it's the most beautiful thing. There are so many people out there who eat a raw diet who are looking for people who eat as they do. To anyone having trouble finding them, I would say, keep searching. Trust me, they are out there. I wish I had a clone, there are just so many.

Do you think it's harder for a woman to eat a raw diet than it is for a man?
It depends. I think emotionally, it is harder for a woman. Physically, I think it's harder for a man. I think women are more emotional eaters, and that might create challenges for them that some men might not have to deal with. I say some men, because I know many men who also emotionally eat. I just see it much more in women. Men, on the other hand, have a hard time because they lose so much weight, and in society they want to look big and strong. Many just don't feel they can be big and

strong looking on this diet. I think that's a myth because people think they don't have to exercise as long as they're eating well. I can guarantee: if people change their diets and do exercise, they will look just fine.

Do you think there are more raw men than raw women?
From what I see, there are. But, I know there are many women out there who eat raw. Since it's harder emotionally for them to do so, I think the rewards are greater. The harder you work, the more appreciation for what you do. There is nothing more beautiful in this world than a woman who eats a raw food diet.

Do you think it's natural for a woman not to bleed during her period when on a raw diet?
I've heard about this and have read books about this topic. I would say it could be natural, but it could also mean a woman is not eating enough fat in her diet or is exercising too much. It could also mean many other things might be wrong. But, a woman in good health will see less of a blood flow than a sick woman. Sometimes they will see no blood flow. Yes, I feel it is natural, as long as that person is in good health.

Do you have any comments about pregnancy and the raw diet?
Just because a woman is not bleeding doesn't mean she's not ovulating. She could be ovulating despite no blood flow, and she could get pregnant. I know a few women who are raw and have gotten pregnant and say there was no discomfort at all. All of them thought out their pregnancy all the way up to the birth of their newborn. Many of these women chose natural childbirth methods instead of going to the hospital. I think that is a better choice. I just mentioned that the most beautiful thing in the world is a woman who eats a raw food diet. Well, I would like to add to that: the most beautiful thing in the world is a raw couple that has a raw baby. The natural way of course: bringing them up in a natural lifestyle and homeschooling them. What could

be more beautiful than that?

Thank you for giving this interview. Is there anything you would you like to add?
I just want to add that many people have been putting junk into their minds and bodies for a long time. It will take a lot of work to get better. It won't just happen overnight. But it is well worth embarking on a raw diet. It's not just a physical change that you will go though, but a mental change as well. So, be ready. A great way to start is to get rid of your television set. The moment you stop watching television programming, you're taking a big step in the right direction. There are no limits to what you can achieve. Just relax, visualize and believe, and you will get there. Keep moving forward, keep seeking raw knowledge and have a great raw life!

CONCLUSION

Here is an e-mail, written by George Carlin, that was sent to me. About our times, it really says it all. From this e-mail you will see that something is wrong. Isn't it time we wake up? It's time we grow up.

A wonderful message by George Carlin:

"The paradox of our time in history is that we have taller buildings, but shorter tempers, wider freeways, but narrower viewpoints. We spend more, but have less. We buy more, but enjoy less. We have bigger houses and smaller families, more conveniences, but less time.

We have more degrees but less sense, more knowledge, but less judgment, more experts, yet more problems, more medicine, but less wellness.

We drink too much, smoke too much, spend too recklessly, laugh too little, drive too fast, get too angry, stay up too late, get up too tired, read too little, watch TV too much, and pray too seldom. We have multiplied our possessions, but reduced our values. We talk too much, love too seldom, and hate

Conclusion

too often.

We've learned how to make a living, but not a life. We've added years to life not life to years.

We've been all the way to the moon and back, but have trouble crossing the street to meet a new neighbor. We've conquered outer space but not inner space. We've done larger things, but not better things. We've cleaned up the air, but polluted the soul. We've conquered the atom, but not our prejudice. We write more, but learn less. We plan more, but accomplish less. We've learned to rush, but not to wait. We build more computers to hold more information, to produce more copies than ever, but we communicate less and less.

These are the times of fast foods and slow digestion, big men and small character, steep profits and shallow relationships. These are the days of two incomes but more divorce, fancier houses, but broken homes. These are days of quick trips, disposable diapers, throwaway morality, one night stands, overweight bodies, and pills that do everything from cheer, to quiet, to kill. It is a time when there is much in the showroom window and nothing in the stockroom. A time when technology can bring this letter to you, and a time when you can choose either to share this insight, or to just hit delete.

Remember, spend some time with your loved ones, because they are not going to be around forever. Remember, say a kind word to someone who looks up to you in awe, because that little person soon will grow up and leave your side. Remember, to give a warm hug to the one next to you, because that is the only treasure you can give with your heart and it doesn't cost a cent.

Remember, to say, "I love you" to your partner and your loved ones, but most of all mean it. A kiss and an embrace will mend hurt when it comes from deep inside of you. Remember to hold hands and cherish the moment for someday that person will not be there again. Give time to love, give time to speak and give time to share the precious thoughts in your mind."

Conclusion

This e-mail by George Carlin says so much. When I read it, it reminds me of one of the lessons I've learned over the years that has helped me so much. That lesson is: "Less is more." This lesson I first realized when I read *Steps Toward Inner Peace* by an amazing lady named Peace Pilgrim. Her books have really changed my life. As people I know are trying to get more, more, more, I'm working very hard to have less, less and less. As she put it, "you should never want more than you need." When I first heard that, I thought it didn't make sense. I asked myself what about the things that make life easy and fun? Well, the more I thought about it, the more I realized all those things I bought that were supposed to make my life better and more fun, did so only for a short while. But then, as the novelty wore off, they became a burden to me. Before I knew it, I had a house full of stuff. I won't say junk, because someone else sure could have used the stuff. But I had no need for these things. But since I was brought up to think I needed more, more, more, I kept them. From a physical point, all they did was collect dust, but from a mental point, they really kept me from being free and growing.

Look around your house. Do you have anything in your house that you haven't used in the last year? How about the last two years, or five years? Most people do. If you really want to feel amazing and free, give it away to someone who can use this stuff and free yourself of the burden. You might not think having so much stuff is a burden, but as you get rid of it, you'll see what I mean.

The more I grow spiritually, the less I need in life and the happier and freer I am. In every aspect of life, this is true. I've visited houses where one person lives with five bedrooms plus many more rooms. I could live in a room half the size of his bathroom and be happy.

People say that is just a lifestyle difference. Yes, it sure is. My life is free and happy, while their lives are trapped. They're not free. Peace Pilgrim says in her books: "The more stuff you

Conclusion

have, the less you own your stuff and the more your stuff starts to own you." That is so true.

There are many books about living a simple life. People have to understand that there is a big difference between not having something and not wanting something. If someone is homeless because they feel they have no choice, that can be a bad thing. However, if someone is homeless because he chooses to have less and doesn't need a big house because he doesn't have a ton of stuff to keep in it, that's a great thing. He's free to go where he wants, when he wants. When many people hear of the homeless, they think of a bum who smells very bad, who is crazy and has no money. Even many of these homeless people have better health and are for sure much freer than many people with big homes who are slaves to their jobs and their lifestyles. But, just because you're homeless doesn't mean you have to be dirty, crazy, or have no money. You can be very clean, healthy and even have a lot of money. I always kid and say, the people with the biggest houses in the world are the homeless, because their houses are not confined by walls and roofs. I'm not suggesting that people should be homeless. I'm suggesting that people should reevaluate their priorities. The more you have, the less you have. It's such a hard lesson to understand, until you live it.

About the same time I was reading the book by Peace Pilgrim, I met a very wise man who just confirmed the message to me. This man was so free and full of life. I asked him his secret and he told me: "A person should never need more than the amount of stuff that could fit into two suitcases." I'll never forget that lesson and how happy and free that man seemed to be.

Here is a wonderful message from Peace Pilgrim:

Just after I dedicated my life to service, I felt that I could no longer accept more than I need while others in the world have less than they need. This moved me to bring my life down to need level. I thought it would be difficult. I thought it would entail a great many hardships, but I was quite wrong. Instead of hardships, I found a wonderful sense of peace and joy, and a conviction that unnecessary possessions are only unnecessary burdens.

You chose the life you live. No other person makes you get up and go to work all day. No other person makes you hang out late all night drinking, or staying up late at night eating and watching television. The only person that makes you do those things is you. If you think differently, you're just making an excuse to continue doing those things.

When many of us think of the homeless, we think of someone who does drugs or drinks. These people chose to live that life for themselves. To follow is what Peace Pilgrim wrote during one of her walks across the country:

How inspiring it is to walk all day in the sunshine and sleep all night under the stars. What a wonderful experience in simple natural living... You soon put material things in their proper place, realizing that they are there for use, but relinquishing them when they are not useful. You soon experience and learn to appreciate the great freedom of simplicity.

Now does this sound like the typical homeless bum on the street who chooses to live in a dark alleyway? Or does this sound like a beautiful lady who has freedom and chooses to live her life simply and happily? You have a choice about your life.

If we want to change the world for the future, we must reverse what is being done today. It doesn't work. The best place to start is to change ourselves. How you do anything is how you do everything, so be the best you can be in all areas of your life. Don't settle for anything less than the best! Keep seeking knowledge, keep moving forward and keep growing spiritually, and keep shrinking the amount of unnecessary material stuff you have.

A final note about growth: There is only one form of healthy growth, and that is spiritual growth. No matter how much you achieve in your life, the only way to be happy with yourself is to keep growing spiritually. A good friend of mine, Dr. Fred Bisci, a very wise man, tells me all the time, "There is only one key to success and that is to obtain a spirituality and to keep growing spiritually. It's the only way."

Well how do we obtain spirituality and keep it growing? By overcoming problems and figuring out how to overcome setbacks, that's how. Many people try to avoid problems and run from their setbacks. They think of these as bad. When they run from their problems, they're running away from their opportunities for spiritual growth.

Dr. Bisci once told me something about the body that I will never forget. He said, "The body is always moving forward or backwards. If it's not moving at all, then that is the same as moving backwards. The key it to keep moving forward."

Well, it is the same thing with spiritual growth. You either move forward and grow, or you move backwards prolonging your spiritual growth. You can only grow if you're moving forward.

Many strive for a life of no problems or setbacks. How can one grow this way? By solving problems that are brought to us, or that we create, is moving forward. Without problems, we lose our chance to grow.

It is through solving problems correctly that we grow spiritually. We are never given a burden unless we have the capacity to overcome it. If a great problem is set before you, this merely indicates that you have the great inner strength to solve a great problem. There is never really anything to be discouraged about, because difficulties are opportunities for inner growth, and the greater the difficulty the greater the opportunity for growth.

Problems are learning and growing experiences. A life without problems would be a barren existence, without the opportunity for spiritual growth.

Spiritual growth is not easily attained, but it is well worth the effort. It takes time, just as any growth takes time. One should rejoice at small gains and not be impatient, as impatience hampers growth.

Peace Pilgrim

Life without learning is death.

-Unknown

Information will come and go, opinions will come and go, events will happen and pass, things will grow and die, things are here one day and gone the next, ... but an inspired soul will never fade away nor die; as people grow the soul will glow more and more. Even if people are not there yet, their soul is always there, waiting to shine. It is always there. To make it shine the most, smile and enhance the powers of your mind, body and Soul. There are "NO LIMITS" to what you can achieve.

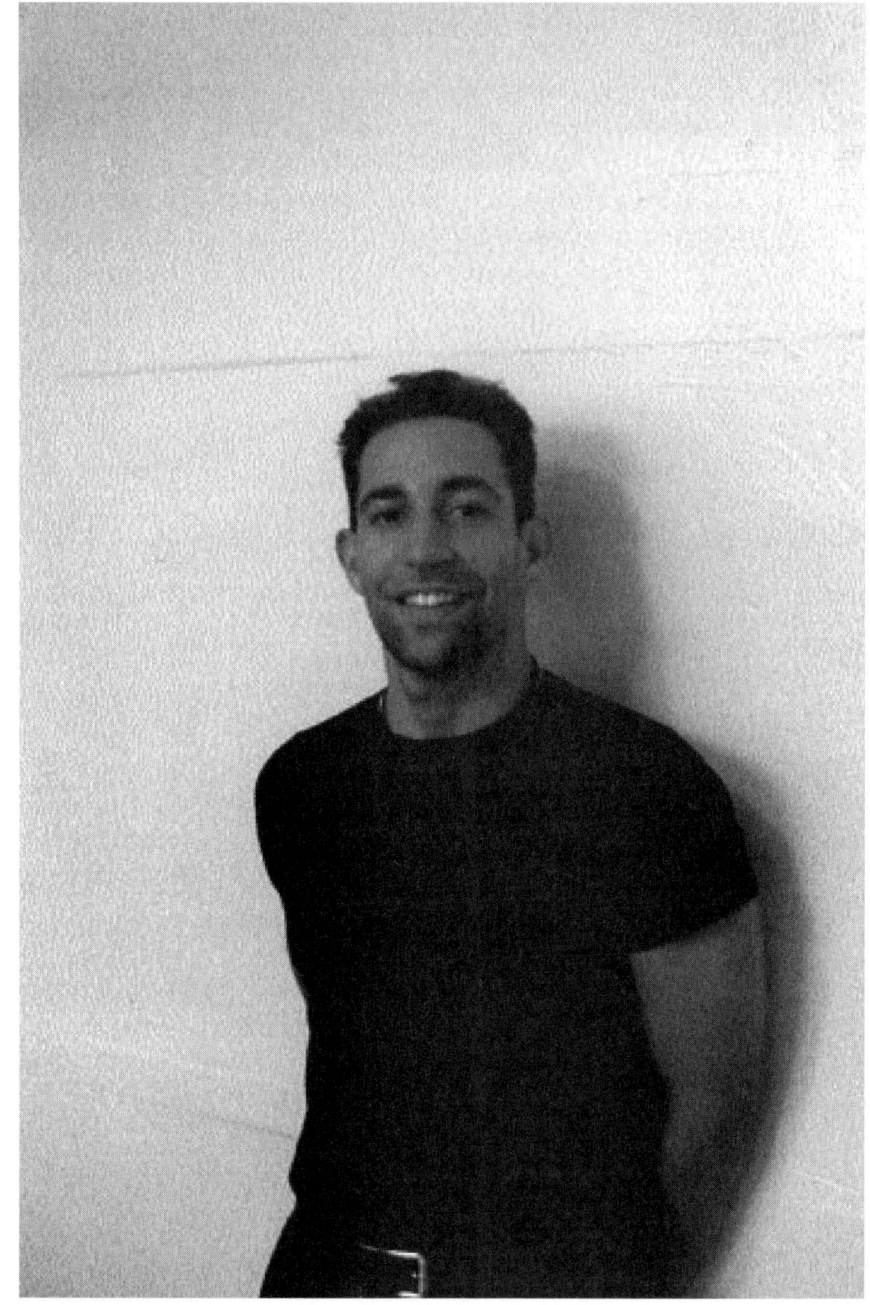

About the Author

Until the age of nineteen, I ate the Standard American Diet (SAD) and never suffered from any problems other than the common upset stomach or headache. Sometimes I would get a cold, but I thought that was normal. But then, the stomachaches started to get worse. I would get colds more often, and I started to worry. I decided to go to the hospital and get checked to see what the problem was. After running many tests, the doctors told me I had food poisoning. They gave me some medication and sent me home. I thought the drugs the doctors gave me would cure me, but during the following three weeks the pains kept coming back worse and worse. They got so bad that I wasn't even able to walk five feet without having to go to the bathroom, whether I had eaten or not. I was wasting away. My weight dropped to 125 pounds, and everyone I knew told me I looked terrible. I tried everything I could think of that would put weight on my body. I ate big portions of fatty foods with increasing frequency. Plus, I stopped doing all exercise in order not to burn too many calories. Nothing I tried worked; my condition just kept getting worse. I was willing to deal with the intense pain, but then one night, I saw blood in my stool. Now, I was really scared. I went to the doctor and the lab ran many tests on me. I felt like some scientific experiment. But, I would have done anything to find out what the problem was, so I could cure it. Up until then, I thought everyone had the common pain I was having. But once I saw blood, I knew the problem was much more serious than I had ever imagined.

Finally, from the doctor, I received my wake-up call. I was diagnosed with ulcerative colitis. Although most people would consider this a tragedy, I consider it one of the best things that

About the Author

---

ever happened to me. When I found out what I had, I remember thinking to myself, "Now I can stop trying to figure out what the problem is, and let the doctors cure me." What a big mistake that was.

First, let me explain what ulcerative colitis is. If you've ever had an ulcer, you know how painful that can be; well, my whole intestinal tract was lined with many ulcers. Ohhhhh! The worst pain in the world, and the only relief was to go to the bathroom many times and sit there for about thirty minutes to an hour. I remember, no matter where the bathroom was, people would knock on the door and ask me if I was okay. I would think, "NO, I'm not okay, I'm very sick," but I never said anything, because who would understand? How many people ever heard of ulcerative colitis or knew what it was? In brief, for those of you who still don't understand what it is, ulcerative colitis is not an easy illness to live with. The colon is achy and inflamed with ulcerations, sometimes with bleeding. It is accompanied by spasmodic and frequent bowel movements. The typical poor diet, increased bowel movements, decreased assimilation of swallowed food, along with drug therapies, all add up to malnutrition and decreased vitality, not to mention misery and a ruined life.

I would get colitis flare-ups about six times a year. Every time I went to the doctor, she told me to stay away from dairy foods until I felt better. Then, she increased the dosage of steroids she was giving me. After a few weeks, when I would feel better, she said it was okay to eat dairy foods again. I then ate foods that contained huge amounts of dairy. Sometimes this would be a whole big pizza. Then the flare-ups came back. Finally, I recognized the pattern and cut out dairy products altogether. I was very pleased with the results. I became sick less often. After that, I began to eliminate whatever the doctors told me it was okay to eat: eggs, meat and sugar to name just a few. I told my doctor, "I feel better without these foods."

She told me, "Food has nothing to do with your condition."

About the Author

After hearing that from her, I knew I was on the right track. I said to myself, "If she's such a good doctor, why do I keep seeing the same people in the waiting room every time I come for a visit? She doesn't heal them, that's why. If she did, they wouldn't need to come back."

At age twenty-three, I left my stressful job as an office manager for a big Wall Street firm in New York's financial district, and moved to West Palm Beach, Florida. I was still having colitis flare-ups, but not as often or severe. By seemingly sheer coincidence, I moved near a place called the Hippocrates Health Institute. I would visit the Institute often during my daily walks around the neighborhood. It was there that I learned about the raw-food lifestyle and about live foods. I immediately put myself on an 80% raw-food diet. What a difference it made! I told my doctor in New York about my improvement and she said, "Raw foods are no good for your condition." Once again, I knew I was on the right track!

Feeling much better, but not totally cured, when I was 25, I moved back to New York and resumed working at the stressful job I had left. In New York, I met many people who had adopted a raw-food diet. I began reading books on the raw-food diet and lifestyle. In a Manhattan bookstore, I picked up a book by David Klein called, *The Fruits of Healing, - A Story about a Natural Healing of Ulcerative Colitis*. It was exactly what I needed to read. I then heard David Wolfe, of Nature's First Law, speaking on a local radio show about the raw-food diet. Nature's First Law is an organization dedicated to spreading the word about the raw food movement. David Wolfe is one of the authors of *Nature's First Law: The Raw Food Diet*, a book he and his co-authors wrote. After speaking to Dave Klein and hearing David Wolfe on the radio, I decided to switch to a 100% raw-food diet. I also decided to join a raw-food support group. At that support group, I met raw foodists, Matt Grace and Tom Coviello, and later, at a fantastic lecture she gave, I met Roe Gallo. The more I got in-

About the Author

volved with the raw-food lifestyle, the more positive my outlook on life became. Speaking to all of these people, and seeing what great health they enjoyed, influenced me to enjoy a diet consisting mostly of fruit. That was the final piece in my health puzzle.

Since going 100% raw, I have completely overcome ulcerative colitis. I feel better than ever, and have become increasingly inspired about life. I quit my stressful job and began working as a raw-food chef in a vegetarian restaurant. I organize raw-food potlucks every month. I've started a raw-food support group, and I give lectures on the raw-food lifestyle to help others who have gotten their wake-up calls.

I've been traveling the world to experience the pleasures of new cultures and exotic fruits. Since adopting the raw-food diet, I've gone through several "healing crises." I'm happy for these episodes of elimination, as they are clearly my body's way of cleaning, healing and rejuvenating. At one time, my weight went all the way down to 118 pounds, but by then I had gained an understanding of how the body works, and I didn't panic. Now my weight remains at a healthy looking 145 pounds, and I know the raw-food diet is the best way for me to go. The people I knew before I was sick, when I was growing up and overweight, look at me now and tell me I'm too skinny or I'm underweight. But everyone meeting me now, and not knowing me then, tells me how great I look. Either way, I go by how I feel, and I feel great. I think I look great too, and I no longer worry about what other people think. That is another advantage of the raw food diet: I stopped trying to please everyone else, and now I please myself first.

Anyone can overcome any dis-ease or sickness the way I did. My books, videos, tapes, CDs and lectures will help you accomplish that. All I can do is tell you about it, the rest is up to you. I encourage you to learn from my experiences and the experiences of others. With a healthy mind, you can overcome anything.

About the Author

For more information about me, please visit my website at: **www.paulnison.com**

I give lectures all over the world about health and empowerment. To see an updated list of where I will be speaking, go to my website: **www.rawlife.com**. If you would like to have me speak to your group, or if you know someone who might be interested in having me speak, please contact me at the telephone number below.

I'm looking forward to meeting everyone interested in enhancing the powers of his or her mind, body and soul.

You may contact me by telephone at:
866-raw-diet (866-729-3438).

Raw Support: Support the Raw Life

For years I've been on the road giving lectures, spreading the word about the raw food lifestyle, keeping a positive attitude and striving to help you reach your maximum potential in all areas of life. In my talks, I always say that it all comes down to helping yourself first, but giving support to others doesn't fall far behind. What you give is what you get. The more support I give to people, the more support I receive in return. Sometimes I test this theory: I'll give a book away for free, and then someone will buy two books. It really does work.

I love doing what I do: helping people help themselves. Nothing will stop me from living my passion, continuing to lecture and write. As I learn, I grow. The more I grow, the more I see myself changing and becoming that better person I want to be.

I want to thank you for buying this book. I would like to ask you to keep supporting me and the raw food lifestyle and invest in my other writings, audios and videos. Also it would be great if you could invest the time to come to my lectures when I am in your town.

You can view all my items at my website **www.rawlife.com** at that site you can also view my current lecture dates. You may also write to me at the address below for more information.

Thank you and have a great raw life.

Paul Nison, P.O. Box 443, Brooklyn, NY 11209

I'm grateful for the time you've taken to read this book as well as for your support.
Thank You! Thank You! Thank You!

Sincerely,
Paul Nison

*Every second wasted,
Every penny spent unnecessarily,
Every action used without thought
Is keeping you from achieving your goals.
Spend your time cautiously.
Spend your money wisely
And react sensibly.*

*Invest in happiness, freedom and love.
Let there be no such outcome as bad or worse,
Only good and better.
Keep stepping up and always strive for better.
There is no limit to what you can get.
Consistently visualize your dreams.
Believe you will accomplish your goals.
Take action and do not rely on anyone else.*

*Be thankful in advance,
Knowing you will achieve
All the goals you set
And all the dreams you create.*

*They are easy to get,
But only dreaming about them
Will not make them a reality.
Take action and get them.
Keep moving forward
And always go after your dreams
And become the person you are.*

ORDER FORM

RAW KNOWLEDGE: ENHANCE THE POWERS OF YOUR MIND, BODY AND SOUL
PLEASE SEND ME ___ COPIES AT **US$ 24.95 PER COPY**

RAW KNOWLEDGE PART II: INTERVIEWS WITH HEALTH ACHIEVERS
PLEASE SEND ME ___ COPIES AT **US$ 19.95 PER COPY**

THE RAW LIFE: BECOMING NATURAL IN AN UNNATURAL WORLD
PLEASE SEND ME ___ COPIES AT **US$ 19.95 PER COPY**

US Shipping and Handling:
$3.50 per first item, $1.00 for each additional item.
Canada and Mexico Shipping and Handling:
$15.00 per first item, $6.00 for each additional item
Outside North America Shipping and Handling:
$25.00 per first item, $6.00 for each additional item

TOTAL AMOUNT ENCLOSED $_____

SHIP TO:
(Please print)

NAME _____

ADDRESS_____

CITY_____ STATE_____

ZIP CODE_____ COUNTRY_____

EMAIL ADDRESS_____

PHONE NUMBER_____

Please copy or cut out this form and mail with a check, money order or bank draft in US currency payable to:

Paul Nison
P.O. Box 443
Brooklyn, NY 11209

To contact the author, go to the website: www.rawlife.com
You may also call 866-RAW-DIET (866-729-3438)

*As time goes by the mailing address may change several times. Please check website or call for most updated contact information.